Facts and Hopes in Thrombolysis in Acute Myocardial Infarction

International Symposium Aachen
December, 7-8 1985

S. Effert · R. von Essen · P. G. Hugenholtz
R. Uebis · M. Verstraete (Eds.)

Facts and Hopes
in Thrombolysis
in Acute Myocardial Infarction

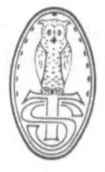
Springer-Verlag Berlin Heidelberg GmbH
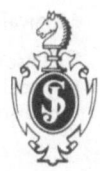

Library of Congress Cataloging in Publication Data.
CIP-Kurztitelaufnahme der Deutschen Bibliothek
Facts and hopes in thrombolysis in acute myocardial infarction: [internat. symposium Aachen, December, 7–8, 1985]/S. Effert... (ed.). – Darmstadt: Steinkopff; New York: Springer, 1986.

ISBN 978-3-662-07176-2   ISBN 978-3-662-07174-8 (eBook)
DOI 10.1007/978-3-662-07174-8

NE: Effert, Sven [Hrsg.]

Medical Editorial: Juliane K. Weller – Copy Editing: Cynthia Feast – Production: Heinz J. Schäfer

Preface

It was a great pleasure for us to welcome so many experts from all over the world to our symposium in Aachen. We are also pleased – and you can attribute this to my own vanity – with the success and acceptance of the concept of myocardial reperfusion and revascularization – specifically selective intracoronary lysis followed either by PTCA or bypass surgery – which we have been pursuing since 1979. But after the dramatic immediate effects of the first attempts, which you have to experience yourself, we did not expect it to be any different. We decided against performing a randomized study in which every patient is catheterized, and thrombolytic therapy only given to some of the patients, for which we have been criticized at times. At the previous symposium in Aachen in 1983 on the topic of thrombolysis for acute myocardial infarction, in the final session several speakers were asked directly about this topic, and replied that if they were patients they would not want to be randomized into the placebo group.

In the meantime positive results from large, randomized studies have been recorded, which are presented in this volume. I mention in particular the Western Washington Study from Dr. Kennedy and the Interuniversity Study in Holland.

Aachen, a relatively small city with 250,000 inhabitants, provided the opportunity to treat a relatively large patient population with acute myocardial infarction. I thank the hospital directors in Aachen and the surrounding area who have made it possible to put together a collection of about 600 thrombolysis patients and 220 with thrombolysis and PTCA. Acute and follow-up angiography have provided important information, not only for the evaluation of thrombolytic therapy, but also on the coronary status of acute myocardial infarction and unstable angina pectoris. We should like to thank Dr. von Essen and Dr. Uebis for organizing the entire symposium. Thanks are also due to all the participants, from 25 different countries, and particularly to the speakers, drawn from seven countries.

The European and American rt-PA Investigation Groups were represented by Professors Verstraete, Passamani and Roberts.

We are grateful to the Companies of Boehringer Ingelheim and Thomae for their support of this conference.

We are pleased that this symposium took place under the auspices of the European Society of Cardiology and the German Society for Heart and Circulation Research, the latter being represented by the president, Professor Bender, and permanent secretary, Professor Schaper.

Aachen, May 1986   S. Effert

Contents

The role of ATP depletion and accumulated metabolic products during myocardial ischemia

J. R. Neely

Milton S. Hershey Medical Center, Pennsylvania, State University, Hershey, PA (U.S.A.)

Introduction

Over the past few years we have directed a considerable amount of effort toward identification of the sequence of biochemical changes which result in a transition of ischemic myocardium from reversibly damaged to irreversibly damaged tissue. For most of the studies that I will describe we have used the isolated perfused rat heart which is exposed to global ischemia. The general protocol that we have followed consists of perfusion of the heart under normal aerobic conditions for a period of 10 min (Fig. 1, top panel). Ischemia, either at zero coronary flow or any reduced flow desired is then instituted for various times and the heart is reperfused for 30 min under normal aerobic conditions. Recovery of ventricular function and restorations of tissue metabolites are followed. If the tissue is reperfused early in ischemia the ventricle will recover metabolically and functionally without much difficulty. It is not surprising, however, that the longer the ischemic period is prolonged, the worse the recovery becomes with reperfusion. The top panel in Fig. 1 shows the change in metabolites and depression of ventricular function after 30 min of zero coronary flow.

Ischemia basically results in two primary alterations of the tissue that may initiate the sequence of changes that lead to irreversible damage. One of these is the loss of oxidative production of high energy phosphate. As a result, total adenine nucleotides and particularly ATP decline during the course of ischemia (Fig. 1). The loss of total adenine nucleotides then prevents the recovery of ATP when the heart is reperfused because there is little ADP and AMP rephosphorylated. The loss of nucleotides is time dependent and at some period of ischemia adenine nucleotides would reach a critically low level and could account for irreversible damage to the cells. The second major problem of ischemic tissue is the accumulation of metabolic products. This is due both to a lack of oxidative metabolism which normally converts the products to CO_2 and H_2O and to a lack of washout of coronary vessels. In Fig. 1, lactate is used as an example of a glycolytic product that accumulates during ischemia. Most of this lactate comes from breakdown of tissue glycogen. These time dependent metabolic changes are associated with the development of a time dependent inability of the heart to recover ventricular function with reperfusion as exemplified by a high diastolic pressure and a low systolic pressure. In the past few years we have attempted to define the specific role of the loss of adenine nucleotides and accumulation of metabolic products in initiating all the other biochemical changes that occur in the tissue that eventually result in the transition from reversible to irreversible damage.

We and many other investigators have found that as the level of total adenine nucleotides decreases during ischemia, mechanical function during reperfusion de-

1

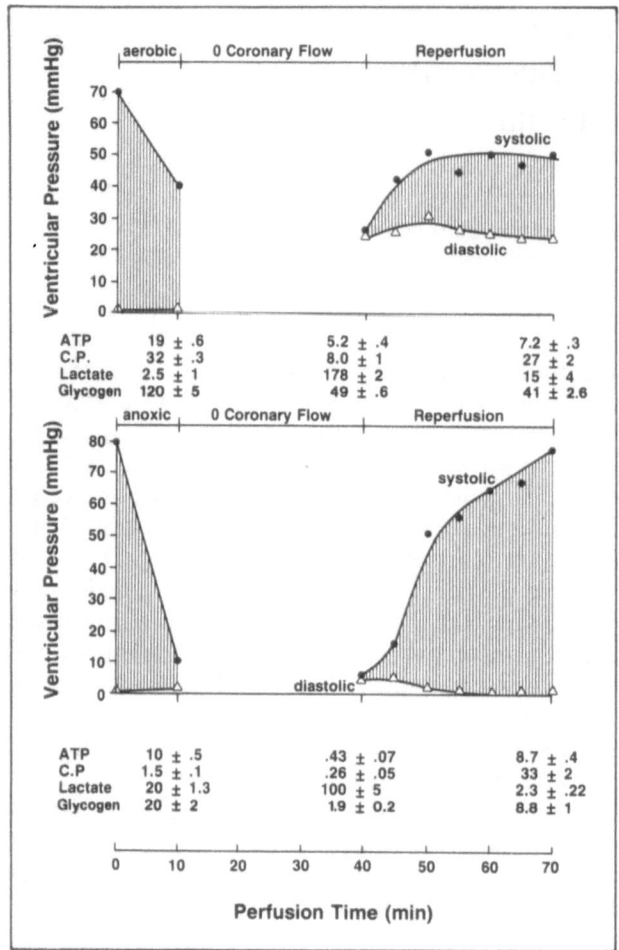

Fig. 1.

clines. When reperfusion function is related to residual ATP levels present during reperfusion, a correlation exists. However, the curve relating these two parameters is not unique. It is influenced by many factors such as Ca^{++} concentration and amount of residual coronary flow during ischemia. The relationship between loss of ATP and loss of mechanical function during reperfusion has been used to argue that the loss of ATP may in fact account for irreversible damage and failure to recover mechanical function with reperfusion. For some years we have proposed that this is probably too simple of an explanation for ischemic cell damage. Other factors are certainly operative. One reason for believing that low ATP is not the only factor initiating damage is that zero recovery of mechanical function occurs when there is still about 2–3 mM ATP left in the cell. This concentration is 10 to 15 times the K_m of the actomyosin interaction for ATP. Another reason for believing that low ATP is not the primary cause of cell damage is that upon reperfusion of ischemic tissue, ATP levels recover very quickly to the extent that ADP and AMP remain. The recovered

ATP, although lower than normal, remains at this new level while ventricular function is depressed. In other words, if ATP levels limited recovery of contractile function, then the ATP level should stay down at the very low ischemic level, not at the higher recovered level. The same is true of creatine phosphate. This suggests that the reperfused tissue is capable of producing ATP and creatine phosphate faster than they are used by muscle and that this is not the contraction rate limiting step in the recovery of function. I would like to now consider the role of metabolic products in cellular damage and to present some data which show more directly that failure to fully recover ATP is not the major problem in reperfused ischemic hearts.

Many years ago we demonstrated that ischemia is a very different process than anoxia. Glycolysis is greatly accelerated in anoxic tissue where flow is maintained but oxygen is removed. However, in severely ischemic tissue glycolysis becomes inhibited secondary to accumulation of glycolytic products (lactate, H^+, NADH). This in itself can account for loss of some of the ATP production during ischemia i.e., the anaerobic production of ATP is much lower. In addition, accumulation of high levels of lactate, H^+, and NADH was associated with depressed recovery of mechanical function. Therefore, we decided to investigate the role of glycolytic products in initiating or accelerating development of cellular damage. To do this, we have used these experimental approaches: glycogen depletion prior to ischemic, maintenance of a low anoxic coronary flow to washout vascular lactate and H^+ and inhibition of glycolysis with 2-deoxyglucose.

Glycogen depletion was produced by perfusion of the hearts for 10 min with a high coronary flow, but with an anoxic perfusate (Fig. 1, bottom panel). Tissue glycogen was broken down during this 10 min period, but very little lactate accumulated due to the high coronary flow. A great deal of the ATP and creatine phosphate was lost during this early anoxic perfusion. When the anoxic perfusion was followed by a period of zero flow ischemia, adenine nucleotide and creatine phosphate were reduced further, almost to zero level or at least to non-detectable levels. These were a great deal lower than in aerobic hearts made ischemic for the same period. Energetically, the glycogen depleted hearts were worse off during ischemia than were the hearts made ischemic with normal glycogen. However, metabolic products during ischemia were less in the glycogen depleted tissue. Also, recovery of ventricular function over 30 min of reperfusion was much better in the glycogen depleted hearts even though ATP and CP recovered to about the same level (Fig. 1). This is another condition where recovery of ventricular function could be dissociated from the residual tissue level of ATP. If lactate, or metabolic products associated with lactate, are detrimental to the ischemic heart, as indicated in Fig. 1, addition of lactate back to the glycogen depleted hearts prior to ischemia should reduce recovery of function with reperfusion. Figure 2 panel A shows the depressed recovery of function during reperfusion of those hearts made ischemic with normal glycogen content. Panel B shows recovery of function in those hearts protected by glycogen depletion and panel C shows that addition of 30 mM lactate to the perfusate during the 10 min anoxic preperfusion prior to ischemia resulted in severely depressed ability to recover ventricular function. The protective effect of glycogen depletion was still very evident when the anoxic perfused hearts were reoxygenated for 10 min prior to ischemia (panel C, Fig. 2). The data in Figs. 1 and 2 strongly suggest that ATP loss is not the primary initiator of irreversible damage to the cell and that it may well be related to the ac-

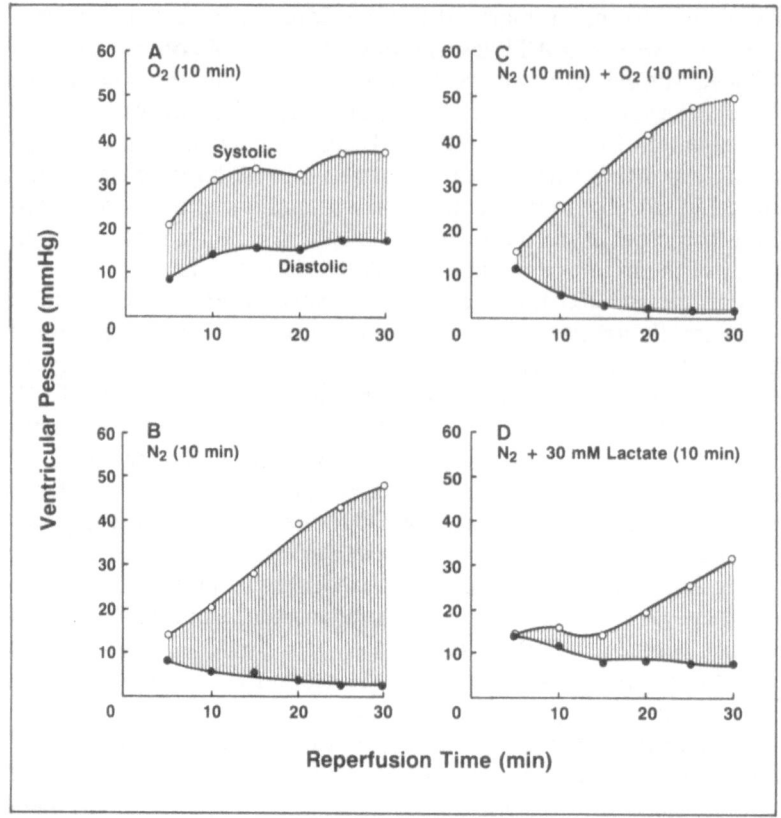

Fig. 2.

cumulation of metabolic products such as lactate or associated metabolites (H^+ and NADH).

Maintenance of a low coronary flow with anoxic buffer also protects the heart compared to those made ischemic with zero coronary flow (Fig. 3). In this study, ATP levels and ventricular function were measured prior to ischemia and at the end of 30 min or reperfusion under aerobic conditions following the times of ischemia shown in the figure. After 30 min of zero coronary flow, recovery of function during reperfusion was about 30% of the preischemic function. ATP levels recovered to only about 7 μmoles/g dry compared to a control value of about 21. When coronary flow was maintained at ml/min with an anoxic perfusate, recovery of function was 90 to 100% of preischemic function for up to 75 min. ATP levels in these hearts were essentially the same as those that did not recover function following zero flow ischemia. Even after 120 min of low flow anoxia, function still recovered better than in the 30 min total ischemic hearts although ATP levels were even lower. These data also show that washout of metabolic products protects the oxygen depleted heart without maintaining higher levels of ATP.

The third experimental approach to determine the effects of glycolytic products involved pretreatment of the hearts for 10 min with 5 mM glucose and 5 mM 2-deoxy-

4

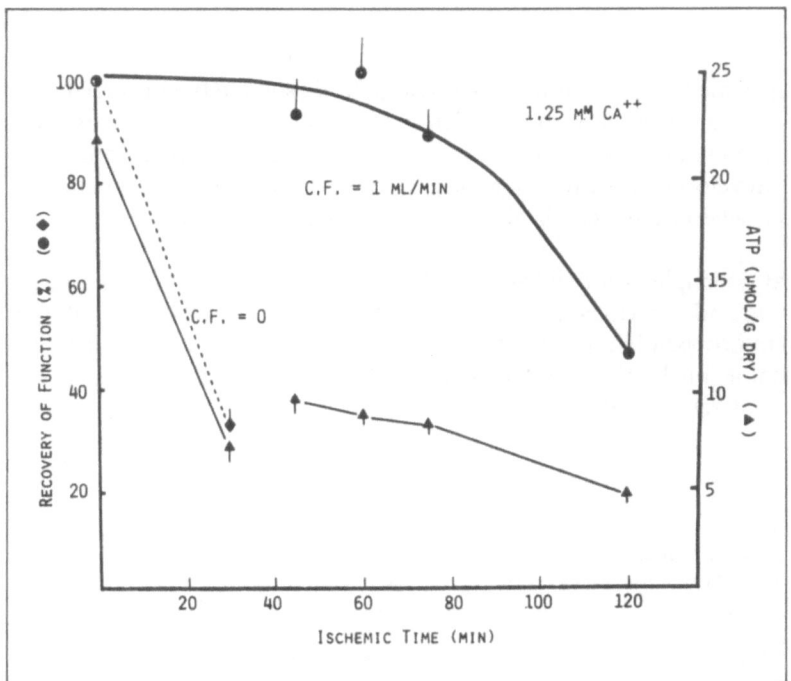

Fig. 3.

glucose prior to exposure to 30 min of zero flow ischemia. In this case, those hearts pretreated with 2-deoxyglucose to inhibit glycolysis had lower levels of lactate, higher levels of glycogen and similar levels of ATP and CP at the end of ischemia compared to untreated hearts (data not shown). During reperfusion, the treated hearts recovered much better ventricular function, but ATP and CP levels were similar to untreated reperfused hearts.

Recovery of ventricular function is rather a crude estimate of cellular damage. However, other parameters such as the well known phenomenon of cellular calcium overload during reperfusion have been used to estimate the degree of cellular damage. Prevention of glycolytic product accumulation during ischemia also greatly reduced the calcium influx during reperfusion in association with improved recovery of mechanical function (data not shown).

If the accumulation of calcium during the reperfusion period is due to lactate or proton induced damage to the tissue during ischemia, addition of lactate to the glycogen depleted heart prior to ischemia should result in an increase in calcium accumulation. This does, in fact, occur. So, here again, adding lactate causes an acceleration of damage as indicated by the accumulation of calcium during reperfusion.

Conclusion

Under certain experimental conditions, it is possible to dissociate the occurrence of cellular damage during ischemia from loss of total adenine nucleotides. The damage is more clearly related to accumulation of metabolic products. However, if one event is prevented, the development of damage may be slowed and thus buy time in the course of ischemia whereby the cell is able to survive and recover function with reperfusion.

It seems clear that no single event will account for the development of cellular damage during ischemia and reperfusion. It is probably better to think of the cumulative effects of several interdependent processes such as accumulation of metabolic products, loss of adenine nucleotides and production of oxygen free radicals as the initiating events that result in damage and cell death.

Author's address:
Professor J. R. Neely
Milton S. Hershey Medical Center
Pennsylvania State University
Hershey, PA 17033
U.S.A.

Ultrastructural aspects of ischemia and reperfusion in canine and human hearts

Jutta Schaper

Max-Planck-Institute, Department of Experimental Cardiology, Bad Nauheim (West Germany)

The ultrastructural analysis of tissue samples from myocardium provides a very precise differentiation of the stages of ischemic injury as well as of the structural recovery occurring during reperfusion of ischemic tissue. A reliable evaluation of the ultrastructural appearance of either ischemic or reperfused human myocardium is only possible after a standardization of all subcellular changes has been carried out under well defined experimental conditions in the dog heart (3). Using the models of both global and regional ischemia followed by reperfusion of the myocardium in the canine heart resuscitability and functional recovery were measured, the content of high energy phosphates and ultrastructural alterations were determined. By comparison of these three independent measurements a "calibration" of the subcellular changes was achieved which allows the exact diagnosis of different degrees of reversible and of irreversible ischemic injury. The following figures show examples of the ultrastructural appearance of normal (Fig. 1) and moderately injured (Fig. 2) myocardium. Figure 3 shows the beginning of structural recovery after moderate ischemic injury, i.e. the beneficial effect of reperfusion. A more detailed description of the changes may be found in the legends of the figures. Table 1 shows the ultrastructural

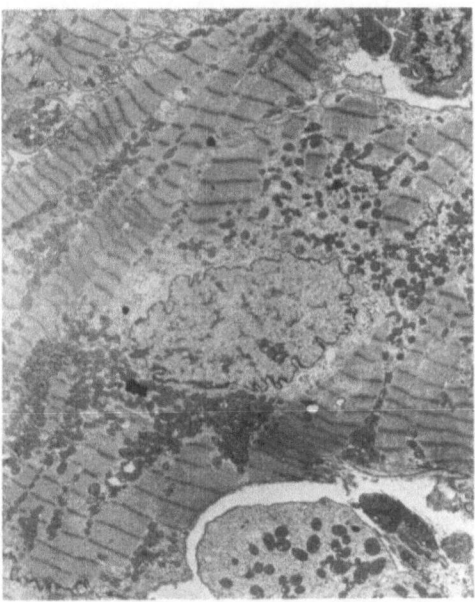

Fig. 1. Nonischemic human myocardium that shows a nucleus with regular chromatin, dense mitochondria, and somewhat contracted sarcomeres. Magn X 1500

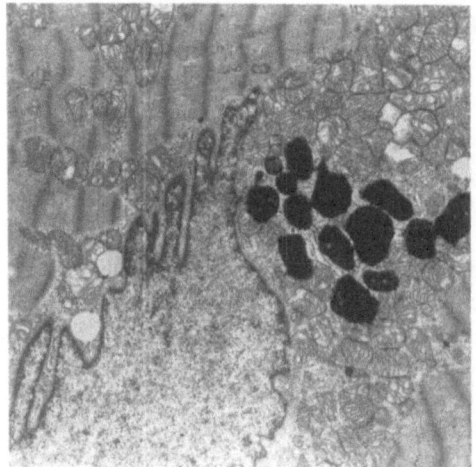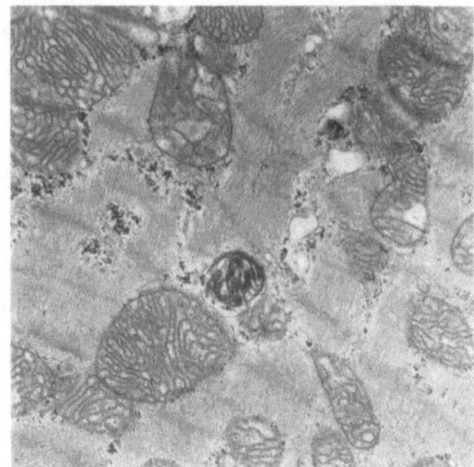

Fig. 2   **Fig. 3**

Fig. 2. Moderate ischemic injury characterized by slight clearing of the nucleoplasm, clearing of the mitochondrial matrix, and fragmentation of mitochondrial cristae. Magn X 3 500

Fig. 3. Structural recovery of mitochondria after moderate ischemic injury. Normal matrix granules begin to reappear, and the mitochondrial matrix is less electron lucent. Magn X 5 000

signs corresponding to different degrees of ischemic injury. This evaluation system is used in daily routine in our laboratory.

In reversible ischemic injury, the ATP content of the myocardium declines significantly and increases only slightly during the early reperfusion period (Fig. 4). Experiments in canine hearts have shown that it may take as long as 4 days until normal ATP levels are achieved again after a 15 min period of ischemia (1). In contrast to reversible ischemic injury, that is, per definition, characterized by a recovery process during reperfusion, irreversible injury represents cell death and leads to necrosis. In this stage of ischemic injury the mitochondria are very electron lucent containing only a few cristae but numerous flocculent densities (Fig. 5). The nucleus shows edema and clumping of the chromatin. Upon reperfusion, the myocardial cells show

Table 1. Typical ultrastructural symptoms in different degrees of ischemic injury in cardiac tissue

State of the myocardium (normal or degree of ischemic injury)	Ultrastructure							
	Mitochondria				Nuclei		Myofilaments	
	Normal granul. + or −	Flocculent densities + or −	Matrix light	Cristae broken	Light	Pycnotic	Contracted or relaxed	Contracture bands + or −
Normal	+	−	−	−	−	−	contr.	+/−
Slight	−	−	+	+	−	−	contr.	+/−
Moderate	−	−	+ +	+ +	+	+	contr.	+
Severe	−	−	+ + +	+ + +	+	+	contr.	+
Irreversible	−	+	+ + +	+ + +	+ +	+ +	relaxed	+ +

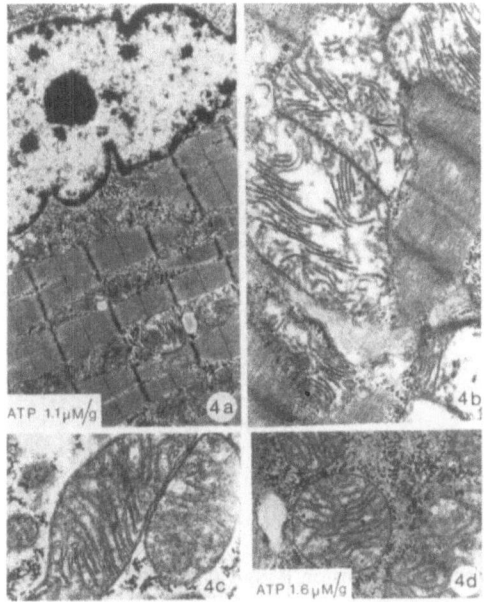

Fig. 4. Severe ischemic injury with low ATP levels (upper panel) that only slightly increase during reperfusion. Mitochondrial recovery, however, is far more progressed (lower panel). Magn X a) 3900, b) 17100, c) 13680, d) 8550

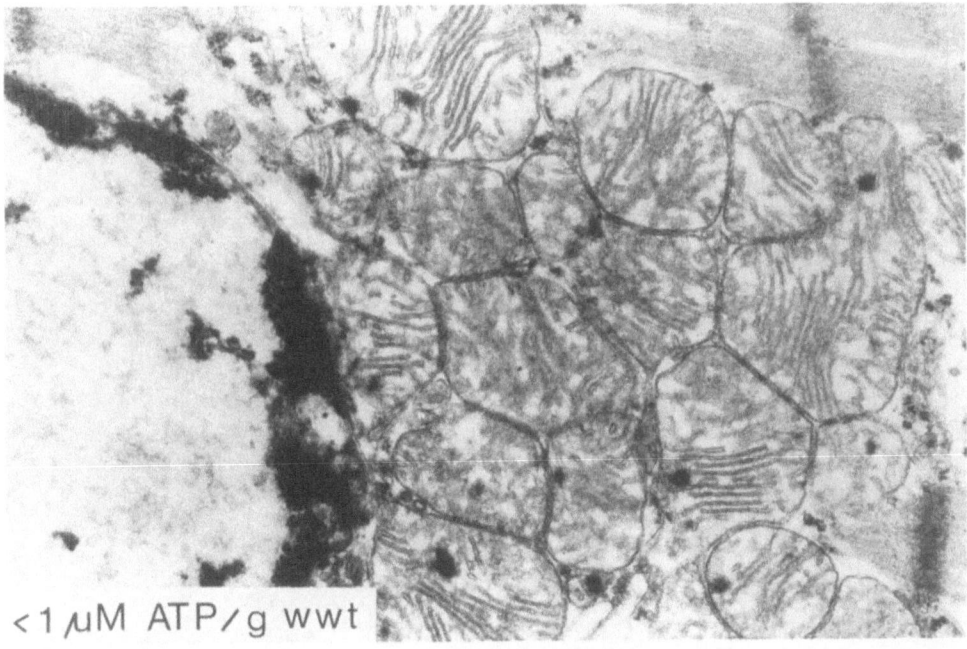

Fig. 5. Irreversible ischemic injury characterized by a cleared nucleus and injured mitochondria that contain flocculent densities. Magn X 31000

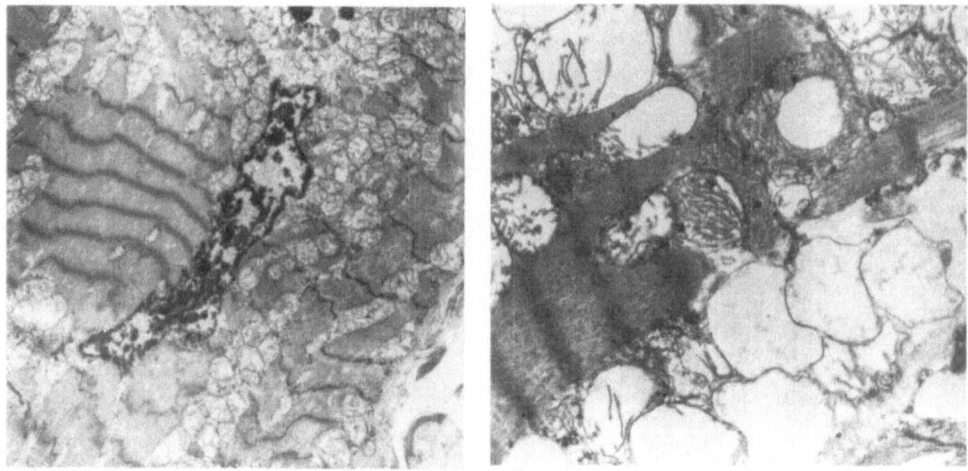

Fig. 6   Fig. 7

Fig. 6. Irreversibly injured myocardium after early reperfusion. Structural damage persists, and contracture bands are evident. Magn X 2 720

Fig. 7. Dissolution of mitochondria during later stages of reperfusion. Magn X 16 500

numerous contracture bands but no structural recovery at all (Fig. 6). Mitochondria and contractile material start to disintegrate and to dissolve (Fig. 7) early after irreversible injury has occurred.

Ischemia affects not only the subcellular structures of the myocytes but those of the microvessels as well. Figure 8 shows the ultrastructural appearance of a normal

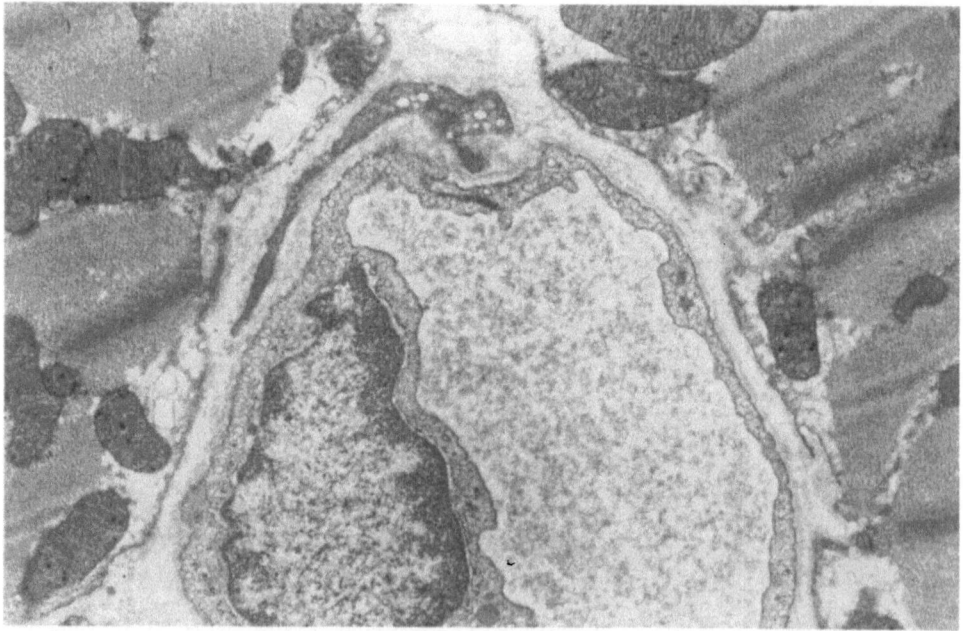

Fig. 8. Normal capillary in the myocardium. Magn X 19 900

10

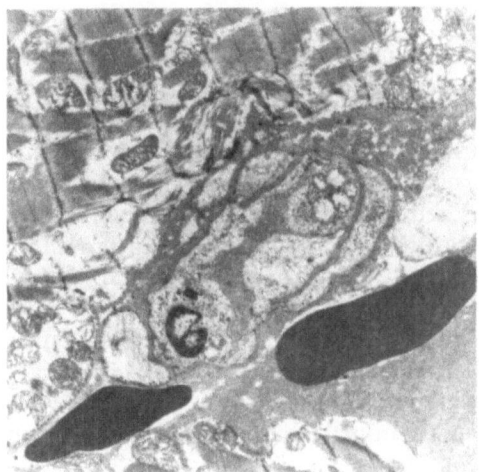

Fig. 9. Capillary in ischemic myocardium showing swollen endothelial cells. Magn X 5 610

capillary and Figure 9 shows a swollen endothelium of a microvessel as observed in reversible ischemic injury. In irreversible injury, the capillaries very often show extensive endothelial swelling or they exhibit complete disintegration. In reversible ischemic injury, the number of swollen endothelial cells of microvessels does not increase upon reperfusion, and the no-reflow-phenomenon is absent (4). A similar situation is present in ischemic and in reperfused human myocardium (5). Reversibly

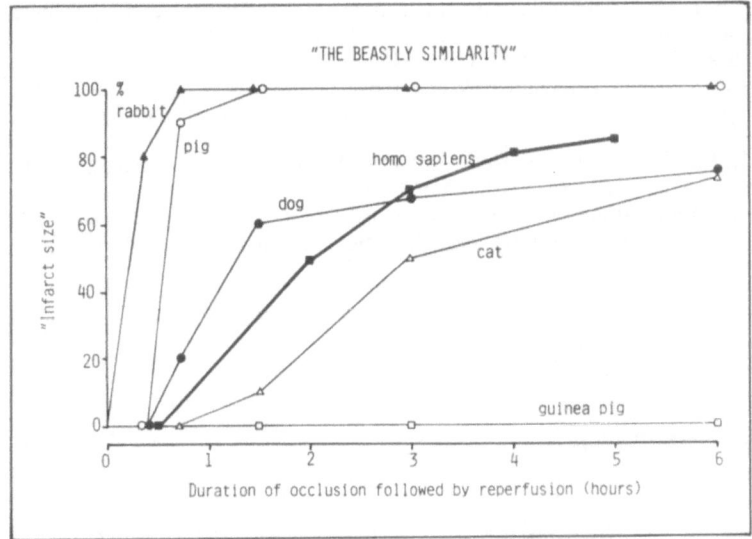

Fig. 10. Infarct size expressed as percentage of the area at risk versus time of occlusion. Rabbits and pigs show early infarction, dogs, humans, and cats show a delayed occurrence of myocardial necrosis, and guinea-pigs do not develop infarction at all. All animal data are from our own studies (6), the human data were obtained in the Thoraxcenter Rotterdam, The Netherlands (courtesy of Professor P. Hugenholtz)

11

injured cardiac tissue is able to recover upon reperfusion, either after global ischemia as used in cardiac surgery or after thrombolysis via catheterization. The ultrastructural appearance of human cardiac tissue reperfused by lysis was characterized by a mixture of reversibly and irreversibly injured cells. Furthermore, intracellular edema was often observed, and hemorrhage and infiltration of leucocytes were common. Several explanations of these ultrastructural findings are possible: the coronary artery may have been only partially opened, or it may have restenosed recently thereby again causing ischemia of the myocardium and subcellular injury to all its components. Where irreversible injury of longer existence had been observed, thrombolysis may have occurred too late, i.e. tissue already irreversibly injured may have been reperfused. It is evident that the time of ischemia plays a decisive role, but it is difficult to determine the absolute time during which salvage of ischemic myocardium is possible. Figure 10 shows species differences, especially differences in the duration of ischemia that causes infarction. Data for human hearts may vary even more than indicated in the figure.

There is no doubt, however, that reperfusion is the only procedure capable of salvaging ischemic myocardium (2).

References

1. Reimer KA, Hill ML, Jennings RB (1981) Prolonged depletion of ATP and of the adenine nucleotide pool due to delayed resynthesis of adenine nucleotides following reversible myocardial ischemic injury in dogs. J Mol Cell Cardiol 13:229–239
2. Schaper J, Schaper W (1983) Reperfusion of ischemic myocardium: ultrastructural and histochemical aspects. J Am Coll Cardiol 1:1037–1046
3. Schaper J, Mulch J, Winkler B, Schaper W (1979) Ultrastructural, functional, and biochemical criteria for estimation of reversibility of ischemic injury: A study on the effects of global ischemia on the isolated dog heart. J Mol Cell Cardiol 11:521–541
4. Schaper J, Schwarz F, Kittstein H, Kreisel E, Winkler B, Hehrlein FW (1980) Ultrastructural evaluation of the effect of global ischemia and reperfusion on human myocardium. Thorac Cardiovasc Surg 28:337–342
5. Schaper J, v Essen R, Messmer B, Effert S, Hehrlein F (1985) Effect of ischemia and reperfusion on myocardium from patients with coronary heart disease. Bibl Cardiol 39:3–13
6. Schaper W (1984) Experimental infarcts and the microcirculation. In: Hearse DJ, Yellon DM (eds) The Approaches to Myocardial Infarct Size Limitation. Raven Press, New York, pp 79–90

Author's address:
Jutta Schaper, M.D.
Max-Planck-Institute
Department of Experimental Cardiology
Benekestrasse 2
D-6350 Bad Nauheim
West Germany

Pro-urokinase and tissue-type plasminogen activator

D. Stump

Center for Thrombosis and Vascular Research, University of Leuven (Belgium)

In this paper I would like to emphasize the mechanisms of fibrinolysis to provide a basic understanding of the events which occur during the lysis of a thrombus in a coronary artery, a deep vein, a pulmonary artery or elsewhere. The key to this process is the conversion of the circulating proenzyme plasminogen to its active enzyme plasmin, which can biochemically dissolve fibrin into fibrin degradation products. Stimulation of this generation of plasmin occurs via plasminogen activators. Those most widely known today are streptokinase and urokinase, tissue-type plasminogen activator or t-PA, single chain urokinase-type plasminogen activator or scu-PA, formerly known as pro-urokinase, and also acylated plasminogen-streptokinase complex. Soon a third generation of these agents will likely be added, consisting of fibrin-specific monoclonal antibodies linked to currently known plasminogen activators, hybrid forms of these natural activators, or new mutations of them. The final molecular component of this system is α_2-antiplasmin, important because it is the most sensitive marker for fibrin specificity.

Fibrin specificity

Plasminogen activators exert their stimulatory effect on the generation of plasmin in two separate compartments. One is in the fluid phase, i.e., in plasma. Here freely circulating plasma is undesirable, although normally it is neutralized very rapidly by the inhibitor α_2-antiplasmin. If plasmin, e.g. during thrombolytic therapy with non-fibrin-specific agents, circulates in the free form, rapid degradation of certain coagulation factors, including fibrinogen, factor V, and factor VIII, occurs leading ultimately to a systemic anticoagulant effect. In contrast, if plasminogen activation were to occur at the fibrin surface, there would exist the possibility for specific degradation of fibrin without release of free plasmin into the circulation. Thus "fibrin specificity" indicates the ability of a given plasminogen activator to stimulate the conversion of plasminogen to plasmin at the fibrin surface and not in the fluid phase (plasma). With an increase in fibrin specificity the potential for clot selectivity is enhanced. Thus, one would like to see optimal fibrin specificity, that is an increasing rate of plasminogen activation occurring at physiological plasminogen concentrations in the presence of fibrin but not in its absence.

Plasminogen and α_2-antiplasmin

One of the key components of this system is plasminogen, the naturally circulating substrate for plasminogen activators. It is a glycoprotein, molecular weight 92,000, activated by the cleavage of a single ARG-VAL bond, yielding a trypsin-like serine protease composed of two polypeptide chains joined by two disulfide bonds. On its structure are lysine binding sites, which are vital for interaction with fibrin and for interaction with α_2-antiplasmin. They are structurally related to the so-called kringle sites, which are important for the natural tendency of plasminogen to interact with fibrin. This places the substrate for fibrinolysis at the fibrin surface, where plasminogen activation can be localized and where the potential of fibrin specific thrombolysis is enhanced (28).

Another key component, α_2-antiplasmin, is a very rapid inhibitor of circulating plasmin which exists to prevent the systemic degradation of coagulation factors by free plasmin. It reacts very quickly with plasmin at an almost diffusion controlled rate, thus being one of the most rapid inhibitory interactions known. However, when plasmin is near the fibrin surface bound via its lysine binding sites, its active site is protected from α_2-antiplasmin and exposed only to fibrin. There its interaction with α_2-antiplasmin only occurs very slowly. Thus nature provides a physiological mechanism for fibrin specific thrombolysis. Ideally one would also seek plasminogen activators which would exert their effects near fibrin, allowing this process to occur only on the fibrin surface. After total lysis, the lysine binding sites of plasmin would be unoccupied, which would then permit rapid interaction with α_2-antiplasmin and inactivation in freely circulating plasma (2).

t-PA

Two new second generation thrombolytic agents have now been identified, specifically t-PA and pro-urokinase (scu-PA). t-PA is fairly well known. It is a single chain glycoprotein with a molecular weight of 70,000, a trypsin-like serine protease occurring in single chain and two chain structures, both of which are fully active. In addition, it displays a high binding affinity for fibrin (21). Kinetically, in the absence of fibrin, t-PA has a very weak affinity for plasminogen. For an enzyme to react with its substrate, efficient generation of the active enzyme is dependent on two factors. One is the tightness of the interaction between the enzyme and its substrate, or affinity (low K_m). The second is the efficiency, once the interaction has occurred, with which the reaction proceeds, or turnover (high k_{cat}). For t-PA, in the absence of fibrin, it reacts only very slowly with plasminogen due to a high K_m, or low affinity. Therefore, very little plasminogen activation will occur. From the measurement of this affinity it is known that in plasma very little plasminogen activation will occur with physiological levels of t-PA. In fact, studies show that in the presence of fibrin, t-PA has a very high affinity (low K_m) for plasminogen. When t-PA and plasminogen are both bound to the fibrin surface, the conformation of the two molecules then greatly facilitates plasminogen activation (13). The t-PA molecule also contains two disulfide bonded kringle structures similar to those of plasminogen. Evidence is beginning to accumulate that structural elements in this region of the protein may modulate the binding of t-PA to fibrin.

14

Pro-urokinase

Pro-urokinase (single chain precursor form of urokinase, molecular weight 54,000) is a recently purified form of a previously known plasminogen activator. The urokinase molecule that has been known as a thrombolytic agent since the 1950s is a two chain molecule which cannot induce fibrinolysis without the generation of free circulating plasmin. Therefore, it is associated with consumption of fibrinogen and antiplasmin prior to the degradation of fibrin. As early as 1973 the idea of a latent urokinase-like activity in a cell culture medium was recognized (1). In 1977 a "proactivator" was also identified in kidney cell culture media (19). This "latent" or "pro" form was recently purified as a single chain species from urine (14, 22), plasma (29), and cell culture conditioned medium (9, 15, 16, 18, 23, 25, 30) or also was produced by recombinant DNA expression in E. coli (12).

Because the fibrin binding properties of t-PA were clear, attempts to purify pro-urokinase were made using fibrin celite chromatography. Because of this fibrin-celite binding property, it was inferred that pro-urokinase might well have clot specific or fibrin specific properties. In fact, in vitro (11, 24, 31) and animal (3, 4, 10, 11, 24, 26) studies showed it indeed could induce fibrin specific thrombolysis, a phenomenon also documented in initial studies, in patients with acute myocardial infarction (27).

Mechanism of action of pro-urokinase

The mechanism of action of single chain urokinase has in fact now been shown to be rather distinctive. It was assumed that urokinase in the single chain form might bind to fibrin and exert a fibrin specific thrombolytic effect in a very similar mechanism to that of t-PA. However, in contrast to the high affinity of t-PA for a fibrin clot formed either in buffer or in plasma, single chain urokinase does not bind to fibrin (17, 22, 23). Furthermore, kinetic studies have now shown that single chain urokinase can activate plasminogen directly due to its uniquely high affinity (low K_m) for the natural substrate (5, 17). Therefore, rather than pro-urokinase, the designation single chain urokinase-type plasminogen activator has now been adopted (20).

Because of this surprising property of scu-PA, significant activation of plasminogen would normally be expected to occur in plasma, even in the absence of fibrin. However, when plasma is added in increasing amounts to the system, a concentration-dependent inhibition of the single chain urokinase mediated conversion of plasminogen to plasmin is seen. When analyzed kinetically, this appears to be a competitive type of inhibition. In other words, there is a reversible factor(s) in plasma which prevents the high affinity interaction between pro-urokinase and plasminogen. More importantly, if one adds soluble fibrin to this system a concentration dependent reversal of the inhibitory effect results, in contrast to persistent inhibition with the addition of fibrinogen (17). This reversal effect of fibrin represents a distinctive mechanism for the clot-selective thrombolysis mediated by scu-PA. It contrasts with that for t-PA which binds directly to fibrin where it more efficiently activates plasminogen. In the case of scu-PA fibrin does not interact directly with the enzyme but rather reverses the natural inhibition of plasma. Thus, these constitute two entirely different mechanisms.

Synergism of t-PA and scu-PA

Logically when two plasminogen activators act via different mechanisms, it is possible that they could be synergistic. Studies of this possibility in an in vitro plasma clot model have yielded negative results (6, 17). However, in an in vivo model of rabbit jugular vein thrombosis, a highly significant synergic effect was seen when measuring thrombolysis induced by combinations of t-PA and scu-PA. Equal fibrinolytic response resulted when using less than 50% of the total fractional dose of scu-PA and t-PA in combination. A less significant effect was noted with t-PA in combination with two-chain urokinase, while no significant synergism was seen between scu-PA and two-chain urokinase. With all combinations no consumption of fibrinogen or α_2-antiplasmin occurred (7). This phenomenon has also now been confirmed in preliminary trials in patients with acute myocardial infarction (8).

Conclusion

Three key concepts are pertinent to the understanding of clot-selective thrombolysis. First is the concept of fibrin specificity, that is the ability of fibrin to be lysed by plasminogen activation at the surface of the fibrin clot and not in the freely circulating plasma. Second, the fibrin specificity of t-PA is dependent upon direct fibrin binding of the activator itself to the fibrin surface where more efficient plasminogen activation occurs. Finally, the mechanism of action of single chain urokinase-type plasminogen activator, or pro-urokinase, occurs through fibrin-mediated reversal of the inhibitory effect of plasma on the high affinity interaction between it and its natural substrate plasminogen. These concepts will be of great importance in the construction and application of third generation thrombolytic therapeutic protocols.

References

1. Bernik MB (1973) Increased plasminogen activator (urokinase) in tissue culture after fibrin depositon. J Clin Invest 52:823
2. Collen D (1980) On the regulation and control of fibrinolysis. Thromb Haemostas 43:77
3. Collen D, Stassen JM, Blaber M, Winkler M, Verstraete M (1984) Biological and thrombolytic properties of pro-enzyme and active forms of human urokinase. II. Thrombolytic properties of natural and recombinant urokinase in rabbits with experimental jugular vein thrombosis. Thromb Haemostas 52:27
4. Collen D, Stump DC, Van de Werf F, Jang JK, Nobuhara M, Lijnen HR (1985) Coronary thrombolysis in dogs with intravenously administered human pro-urokinase. Circulation 72:384
5. Collen D, Zamarron C, Lijnen HR, Hoylaerts M (1986) Activation of plasminogen by pro-urokinase. II. Kinetics. J Biol Chem 261:1259

16

6. Collen D, De Cock F, Demarsin E, Lijnen HR, Stump DC (1986) Absence of synergism between tissue-type plasminogen activator (t-PA), single-chain urokinase-type plasminogen activator (scu-PA) and urokinase on clot lysis in a plasma milieu in vitro. Thromb Haemostas (in press)
7. Collen D, Stassen JM, Stump DC, Verstraete M (1986) In vivo synergism of thrombolytic agents. Circulation (in press)
8. Collen D, Stump DC, Van de Werf F (1986) Coronary thrombolysis in patients with acute myocardial infarction by intravenous infusion of synergic thrombolytic agents. Am Heart J (in press)
9. Eaton DL, Scott RW, Baker JB (1984) Purification of human fibroblast urokinase proenzyme and analysis of its regulation by proteases and protease nexin. J Biol Chem 259:6241
10. Flameng W, Vanhaecke J, Stump DC, Van de Werf F, Holmes W, Günzler WA, Flohe L, Collen D (1986) Coronary thrombolysis by intravenous infusion of recombinant single-chain urokinase-type plasminogen activator or recombinant urokinase in baboons: effect on regional blood flow, infarct size and hemostasis. J Am Coll Cardiol 8:118
11. Gurewich V, Pannell R, Louie S, Kelley P, Suddith RL, Greenlee R (1984) Effective and fibrin-specific clot lysis by a zymogen precursor form of urokinase (pro-urokinase). A study in vitro and in two animal species. J Clin Invest 73:1731
12. Holmes WE, Pennica D, Blaber M, Rey MW, Günzler WA, Steffens GJ, Heyneker HL (1985) Cloning and expression of the gene for pro-urokinase in escherichia coli. Biotechnology 3:923
13. Hoylaerts M, Rijken DC, Lijnen HR, Collen D (1982) Kinetics of the activation of plasminogen by human tissue plasminogen activator: role of fibrin. J Biol Chem 257:2912
14. Hussain SS, Gurewich V, Lipinski B (1983) Purification and partial characterization of a single-chain high-molecular-weight form of urokinase from human urine. Arch Biochem Biophys 220:31
15. Kasai S, Arimura H, Nishida M, Suyama T (1985) Proteolytic cleavage of single-chain pro-urokinase induces conformational change which follows activation of the zymogen and reduction of its high affinity for fibrin. J Biol Chem 260:12377
16. Kohno T, Hopper P, Lillquist JS, Suddith RL, Greenlee R, Moir DT (1984) Kidney plasminogen activator: a precursor form of human urokinase with high fibrin affinity. Biotechnology 2:628
17. Lijnen HR, Zamarron C, Blaber M, Winkler M, Collen D (1986) Activation of plasminogen by pro-urokinase. I. Mechanism. J Biol Chem 261:1253
18. Nielsen LS, Hansen JG, Skriver L, Wilson EL, Kalthof K, Zeuthen J, Dano K (1982) Purification of zymogen to plasminogen activator from human glioblastoma cells by affinity chromatography with monoclonal antibody. Biochemistry 21:6410
19. Nolan C, Hall LS, Barlow GH, Tribby ILE (1977) Plasminogen activator from human embryonic kidney cell cultures. Evidence for a proactivator. Biochim Biophys Acta 496:384
20. Report of the meeting of the Subcommittee on Fibrinolysis, San Diego, CA, USA, July 13, 1985. Thromb Haemostas 54:893
21. Rijken DC, Collen D (1981) Purification and characterization of the plasminogen activator secreted by human melanoma cells in culture. J Biol Chem 256:7035
22. Stump DC, Thienpont M, Collen D (1982) Urokinase-related proteins in human urine. Isolation and characterization of single-chain urokinase (pro-urokinase) and urokinase-inhibitor complex. J Biol Chem 257:3276
23. Stump DC, Lijnen HR, Collen D (1986) Purification and characterization of single-chain urokinase-type plasminogen activator from human cell cultures. J Biol Chem 261:1274
24. Stump DC, Stassen JM, Demarsin E, Collen D (1986) Comparative thrombolytic properties of single-chain forms of urokinase-type plasminogen activator. Submitted to Blood
25. Sumi H, Kosugi T, Matsuo O, Mihara H (1982) Physicochemical properties of highly purified kidney cultures plasminogen activator (single polypeptide chain-urokinase). Acta Haematol Japon 45:119
26. Sumi H, Maruyama M, Matsuo O, Mihara H, Toki N (1982) Higher fibrin-binding and thrombolytic properties of single polypeptide chain-high molecular weight urokinase. Thromb Haemostas 47:297
27. Van de Werf F, Nobuhara M, Collen D (1986) Coronary thrombolysis with human single-chain, urokinase-type plasminogen activator (pro-urokinase) in patients with acute myocardial infarction. Ann Intern Med 109:345

17

28. Wiman B (1978) Biochemistry of the plasminogen to plasmin conversion. In: Gaffney PJ, Balkuv-Ulutin S (eds) Fibrinolysis, current fundamental and clinical aspects. Academic Press, London, p 47
29. Wun TC, Schleuning WD, Reich E (1982) Isolation and characterization of urokinase from human plasma. J Biol Chem 257:3276
30. Wun TC, Ossowski L, Reich E (1982) A proenzyme form of human urokinase. J Biol Chem 257:7262
31. Zamarron C, Lijnen HR, Van Hoef B, Collen D (1984) Biological and thrombolytic properties of pro-enzyme and active forms of human urokinase. I. Fibrinolytic and fibrinogenolytic properties in human plasma in vitro of urokinases obtained from human urine or by recombinant DNA technology. Thromb Haemostas 52:19

Author's address:

David Stump, M.D.
Assistant Professor in Medicine
Department of Internal Medicine
University of Vermont
College of Medicine
Given Medical Building
Burlington, VT 05405
U.S.A.

Preliminary clinical results with pro-urokinase

F. Van de Werf

Division of Cardiology, Leuven (Belgium)

The purpose of the present paper is to summarize our experience with pro-urokinase (pro-UK), or alternatively designated single chain urokinase-type plasminogen activator, scu-PA, for coronary thrombolysis.
At present, data are available from a limited number of animals and from six patients with acute myocardial infarction. I will first briefly summarize the results of the dog and baboon studies.

Methods

Pro-UK or scu-PA was administered to six dogs with an hour-old clot, induced with a copper coil, in the left anterior descending coronary artery (1). Intravenous infusion of natural pro-UK at a rate of 10 µg/kg per min for 30 min failed to induce thrombolysis in two dogs, which was only obtained after 8 and 15 min of subsequent intracoronary administration. However, intravenous infusion at the rate of 20 µg/kg per min for 30 min in four dogs induced lysis within 23 min on average, and without any change in fibrinogen of α_2-antiplasmin. Figure 1 shows the plasma levels of

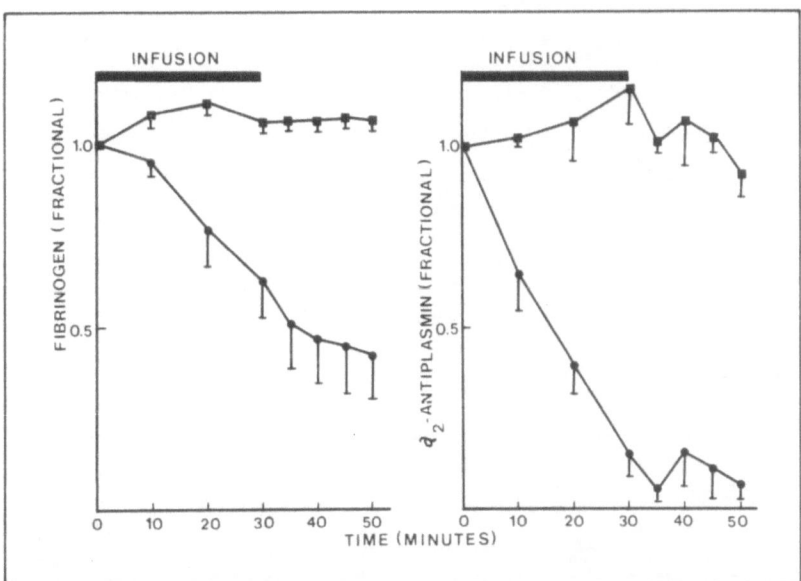

Fig. 1. Changes in fibrinogen and alpha 2-antiplasmin levels in plasma during intravenous infusion of pro-urokinase or urokinase in dogs with acute myocardial infarction. Reproduced from Circulation (1) with the permission of the American Heart Association

fibrinogen and α_2-antiplasmin during infusion of pro-UK and during infusion of equipotent doses of urokinase.

Similar results were obtained in 18 baboons with recombinant pro-UK (2). After intravenous infusion of 20 µg/kg per min for 60 min, complete reperfusion was obtained in all animals after 21 min on average. Also in this species no changes in hemostatic parameters were observed during and after infusion with recombinant pro-UK.

Let us now turn to the patients with acute myocardial infarction. Pro-UK, isolated from the conditioned medium of a human renal adrenocarcinoma, was administered to six patients with an acute infarction of less than 5 h duration. Pro-UK was infused at a rate of 40 mg for 60 min, immediately followed in three of these patients by an intracoronary infusion of 20 mg for 30 min. In all patients, total occlusion of the infarct-related coronary artery was confirmed angiographically prior to the onset of the intravenous infusion.

The average age of the two women and four men was 54 years. Five patients had an inferior and one an anterior myocardial infarction. The time between onset of symptoms and start of infusion ranged between 2.5 h and nearly 5 h. The site of the thrombotic occlusion was the right coronary artery in five patients, and the left main coronary artery in one patient.

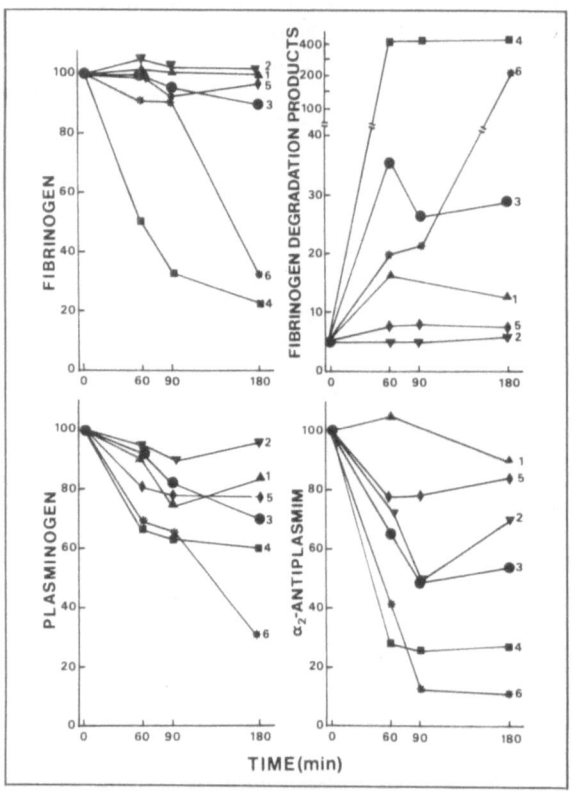

Fig. 2. Changes in hemostatic parameters after infusion of pro-UK. Reproduced with permission from Annals of Internal Medicine (3)

20

Results

Complete lysis was achieved during intravenous infusion in 4 patients (patients 1, 3, 4 and 5) and after 20 min of subsequent intracoronary infusion in one patient (patient 2). The last patient (patient 6) did not respond to pro-UK but was also unresponsive to intracoronary infusion of 250,000 units of streptokinase. Patient 3 received an intracoronary dose of pro-UK despite complete reperfusion after intravenous infusion because of the critical location of the residual stenosis (left main coronary artery).

Pro-UK did not induce an overt systemic lytic state in 5 of the 6 patients (patients 1, 2, 3, 5 and 6) as evidenced by the unchanged levels of fibrinogen and the lack of generation of significant amounts of fibrinogen degradation products (Fig. 2). In one patient (patient 4) the fibrinogen level decreased to about 25% of the infusion level and higher levels of fibrinogen degradation products were observed. The intracoronary infusion of streptokinase in patient 6 was also associated with a hemostatic breakdown which was not observed during the administration of pro-UK (3).

Conclusion

In conclusion, we consider scu-PA or pro-UK to be a clot selective thrombolytic agent capable of inducing coronary thrombolysis without or associated with moderate systemic fibrinolysis in patients with acute MI. Preliminary experience from our studies suggests that scu-PA or pro-UK may constitute an effective and safe intravenous agent for coronary thrombolysis and provides a basis for the design of future controlled clinical trials with recombinant material.

Acknowledgements. Natural pro-UK was provided by Mochida Chemical Co., Tokyo, Japan; recombinant pro-UK was provided by Grünenthal GmbH, Aachen, F.R.G.

References

1. Collen D, Stump D, Van de Werf F, Jong IK, Nobuhara M, Lynen HR (1985) Coronary thrombolysis in dogs with intravenously administered human pro-urokinase. Circulation 72:384–388
2. Flameng W, Vauhaecke J, Stump D, Van de Werf F, Holmes W, Günzler W, Flohé L, Collen D (1986) Coronary thrombolysis by intravenous infusion of recombinant single-chain urokinase-type plasminogen activator or recombinant pro-urokinase in baboons. J Am Coll Cardiol (in press)
3. Van de Werf F, Nobuhara M, Collen D (1986) Coronary thrombolysis with human single-chain, urokinase-type plasminogen activator (pro-urokinase) in patients with acute myocardial infarction. Ann Intern Med 104:345–348

Author's address:
Professor F. Van de Werf
Division of Cardiology
K.U.L. Campus Gasthuisberg
Heerestraat 49
3000 Leuven, Belgium

Anisoylated streptokinase plasminogen activator

R. Vincent

Cardiac Department, Royal Sussex County Hospital, Brighton (U.K.)

Introduction

The advantages of intravenous fibrin-specific agents are well-recognised. They fulfil our aim to achieve a high local concentration of thrombolytic activity with the benefits of relative ease and speed of administration. They may also achieve a low-level systemic effect which may in theory prove beneficial in opposing early arterial reocclusion.

The compound

Figure 1 shows schematically the action of plasminogen, a molecule with potential "jaws". (Thrombosis is clearly seen as an aggressive phenomenon!) Activation of plasminogen opens its "jaws" (Fig. 1 b) to effect lysis at a thrombin site. Kringles, special structural components of the plasminogen molecule, are helpful here in locating this agent for activation on the developing clot.

A molecule of streptokinase can combine with plasminogen causing a conformational change illustrated here as the extrusion of a sharp "point" (Fig. 2). The plas-

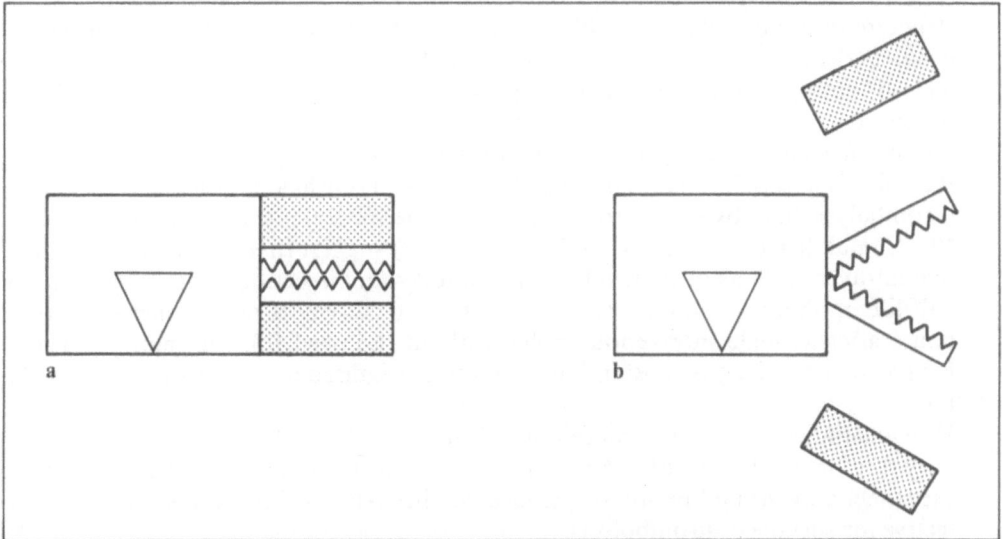

Fig. 1. A schematic representation of a plasminogen molecule in its inactive form (a) and in its activated form for thrombolysis (b). See text

23

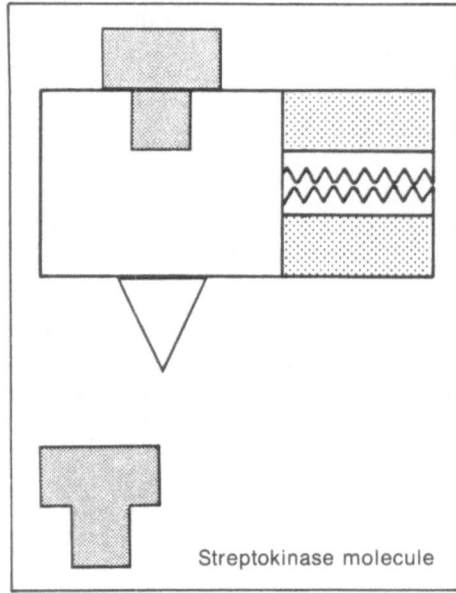

Streptokinase molecule

Fig. 2. A schematic diagram of a plasminogen molecule to which streptokinase has become attached causing a conformational change. See text

minogen-streptokinase complex itself activates further plasminogen molecules opening the "jaws" to initiate thrombolytic activity (Fig. 3). It should be noted that one plasminogen molecule is consumed in this interaction; thus, theoretically, streptokinase in high therapeutic doses could saturate the available plasminogen supply.

In the compound discussed in this paper (BRL 26921) (11) a protective "cover" has been built over the activation "point" of the plasminogen-streptokinase complex (Fig. 4). The anisoyl group which "covers" this site of activation thus completes the structure of a molecule that is fibrin specific but without thrombolytic effect until it has undergone deacylation in vivo. Logically, this compound may therefore be termed "anisoylated-plasminogen-streptokinase-activator-complex" – or "APSAC" for short.

APSAC has been studied in a variety of thrombotic conditions including deep vein thrombosis and pulmonary embolism (3, 8, 11); and it has been used for coronary thrombolysis both by intracoronary (1, 6) and peripheral intravenous delivery (2, 5, 12). Cumulative dose-ranging studies (2, 5, 7, 12) suggest that it is maximally effective intravenously as a single 30 mg bolus; following injection it has a deacylation half-life of about 40 minutes (11). Thrombolytic activity is maintained for several hours after a single intravenous bolus without the need for continuing infusion. Moreover, its activity is substantially if not fully localised to the site of recent thrombosis.

Human studies in a total of more than 150 patients have shown that 87% of coronary thrombi are lysed within 60 minutes of administration of this agent. Thus both experimentally (4) and in invasive clinical studies APSAC has been shown to be effective for sustained thrombolysis.

At the Royal Sussex Hospital in Brighton we have explored the pragmatic use of this agent in the treatment of acute myocardial infarction. Our hospital serves a popu-

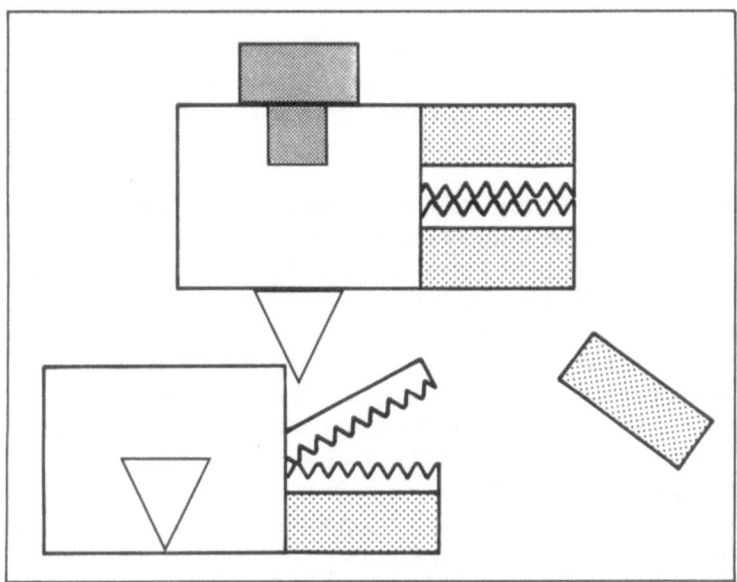

Fig. 3. A schematic representation of a plasminogen-streptokinase complex activating a second plasminogen molecule. See text

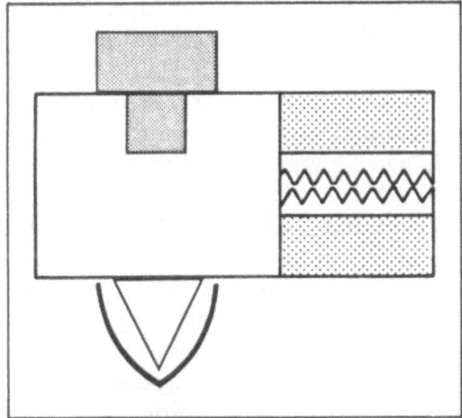

Fig. 4. A schematic diagram showing a plasminogen streptokinase complex in which the activator site has been "covered" by an anisoyl group. This is anisoylated plasminogen streptokinase activator complex – APSAC. See text

lation of about 350 000 and supports a Resuscitation Ambulance Service. As a result of this service the median time for admission of suspected coronary patients has been reduced to about two hours – an advantage for the delivery of thrombolytic agents early in the course of a coronary attack. It was in this setting that we aimed to study the use of APSAC in about 150 patients in an open controlled trial.

Methods

The efficacy of a single intravenous bolus of APSAC early in the course of suspected acute myocardial infarction was assessed by clinical progress and by non-invasive techniques. Special attention was given to the recording of suspected adverse effects.

Patients were suspected of having acute myocardial infarction if they presented with typical cardiac pain lasting for more than 30 minutes and if the electrocardiogram showed ST segment elevation of at least 1 mm. All patients were given glyceryl trinitrate (sublingually or by spray), and only if diagnostic ST segment elevation persisted were they admitted to the trial. Patients in the study population were of either sex and were under 75 years of age. They were divided prospectively into two groups: an early group in which patients were entered within 2½ hours of the onset of major symptoms, and a late group in which the delay to entry was between 2½ and 4 hours. The division at 2½ hours was chosen in the light of a previous analysis of the time of admission of infarct patients in relation to symptoms; from this we judged that a break point of 2½ hours would give us the best opportunity of admitting equal numbers of patients to the early and late entry groups.

During the period of the study – February 1984 to March 1985 – 563 patients with suspected infarction were considered of whom 149 (27%) were admitted to the trial. The main criteria for exclusion were the lack of persistent ECG changes, arrival too late for entry (in spite of the Resuscitation Ambulance Service), and being above the age limit. Other exclusion criteria included cardiogenic shock, bleeding diathesis, and treatment with thrombolytic or anticoagulant therapy in the previous six months. (These latter categories eliminated some of the higher risk patients from our study.)

In the study population, treatment and control groups were comparable for gender, previous infarction, admission blood pressure, and the Norris Coronary Prognostic Index (9). There was a slight difference in mean age between control and treatment groups, being slightly higher in the controls.

As soon as was practicable after admission to the trial patients in the treatment group were given a single 30 mg bolus of APSAC by intravenous injection over 4 minutes. In both groups therapy was continued with a low-sodium antacid and anticoagulation with intravenous heparin (routine practice in our Unit).

Following APSAC injection we monitored all patients as follows: by clinical progress – especially in terms of recurrent pain, haemodynamic status, progression to infarction and mortality; by R wave score (a rather coarse electrocardiographic estimate of myocardial preservation); by CK-MB enzyme release, sampling at 6-hourly intervals for the first 48 hours; and by arrhythmia monitoring for the first 24 hours using the Tracker/Pathfinder II system. We also recorded any adverse effects judged to be associated with the use of APSAC.

Results

i) In hospital

Table 1 shows for the control and treatment groups the numbers of patients progressing to confirmed infarction, and the numbers that developed recurrent pain or that

Table 1. Clinical progression of patients in the first seven days

	Control	APSAC	
Confirmed infarction	67 (92%)	60 (79%)	p<0.05
Recurrent pain	46	36	NS
Death by 7 days	6	3	NS

died in the course of the first seven days in hospital. In the control group 92% of patients developed confirmed infarction compared with 79% in the treated group, a difference significant at the $P < 0.05$ level. No statistical difference was observed in the incidence of recurrent pain or in mortality at seven days though trends were noted that appeared favourable for the treatment group.

R wave scores are listed in Table 2. (In this analysis the higher the score the more myocardium has been preserved.) R wave scores showed that in the early entry group (0–2½ hours) significantly less myocardial damage occurred after thrombolytic therapy than in the control group. Less effect was noted in the late entry group (2½–4 hours) but cumulative totals show overall benefit with those receiving APSAC ($P = 0.03$).

We estimated a number of parameters associated with CK-MB release for patients who went on to develop an established myocardial infarction. Table 3 summarises CK-MB release expressed as the area-under-the-curve. No difference in total enzyme release was observed between any of the study groups, although there was a (non-significant) trend toward an earlier peak in enzyme rise in those receiving active treatment.

Table 4 presents an analysis of cardiac rhythm during the first 24 hours expressed as bursts of ventricular tachycardia of 4–10 beats. The early treatment group showed a 57% incidence of runs of self-limiting ventricular tachycardia which was significantly greater than that observed in the control group (31%, $P < 0.05$). In the late group, and in the study overall, these differences were not as pronounced, though the trends remained similar. The interpretation of these results is open to discussion; but reperfusion arrhythmias are well-recognised, and the increased number of arrhythmias observed *could* have resulted from effective thrombolysis with reperfusion.

In Table 5 we record a summary of the adverse effects of APSAC seen in this study. In keeping with its designation as a fibrin-specific agent, APSAC caused few important adverse reactions from a systemic action. But it was interesting to note that pa-

Table 2. R wave scores for the study population and for the early- and late-entry groups

	Control	ASPC	
0–2.5 h	27	44	p<0.02
2.5–4 h	47	53	N.S.
All	36	48	p=0.03

Table 3. CK-MB release expressed as area under-the-curve for the early- and late-entry groups

	Control	ASPC	
0–2.5 h	1951	1887	N.S.
2.5–4 h	1457	1655	N.S.
All	1783	1805	N.S.

Table 4. Patients showing 4–10 beat runs of ventricular tachycardia for the early- and late-entry groups

	Control	APSAC	
Early	31% (9/29)	57% (20/35)	p < 0.05
Late	47% (16/34)	59% (19/32)	NS
Total	40% (25/63)	58% (39/67)	p < 0.05

Table 5. A summary of definite or possible adverse effects from the use of APSAC

Common	– Bruising
Rare	– Blood streaked vomit
	– Flushing
	– Allergic reactions
One patient	– Shower of emboli (late death)

tients receiving APSAC often had more bruising around venous puncture sites than those who had not received this agent. Important bleeding was rare: one case of blood-streaked vomit was reported, and one patient with haemorrhoids bled during the course of admission. Flushing and allergic reactions were also uncommon, although in one patient an unusual form of lower limb rash occurred (Fig. 5) which lasted for several weeks. The rash – of Heinoch-Schonlein type – was self-limiting and was not associated with any haemodynamic disturbance or other signs of allergy.

One patient with a large anterior infarct presented 36 hours after APSAC with an unusual petechial rash over the lower limbs. This was associated with considerable pain in the buttocks, thighs and calves, and appeared to be due to a shower of emboli causing micro-infarction throughout most of the lower limbs. A massive rise in non-

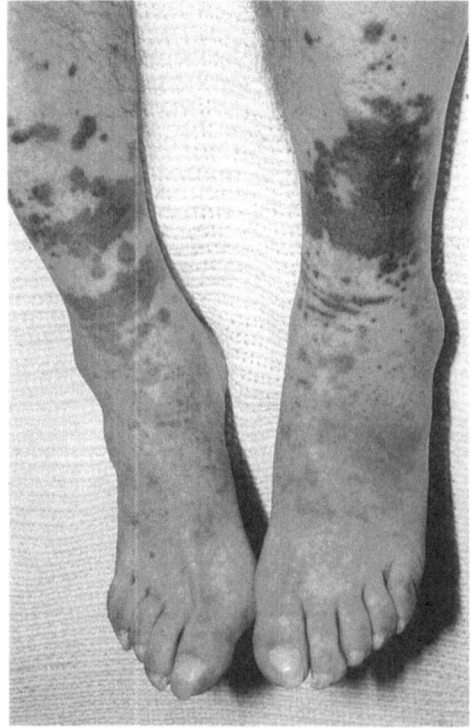

Fig. 5. The Heinoch-Schonlein type rash which developed as an apparent side-effect following APSAC therapy in one patient

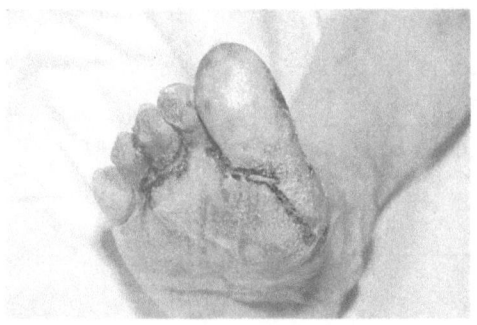

Fig. 6. Gangrene which developed as a result of a shower of peripheral emboli 36 hours after intravenous APSAC

myocardial CK enzyme was recorded and the patient later developed frankly gangrenous feet (Fig. 6). This embolic event was an important contributory factor though not the entire reason for the patient's subsequent death; the infarction itself was large and the patient on first admission had presented with extensive alveolar pulmonary oedema.

ii) Follow-up – preliminary data

We are now close to the end of the follow-up study of this group of patients. Preliminary analysis at a median follow-up time of 10.5 months shows that post-discharge mortality has been universally low; no statistically significant difference has been shown between any of the sub-groups reviewed (Table 6). Though we are still attempting to contact a number of patients who have been lost to follow-up their outcome is unlikely to alter this result.

Follow-up visits have included a non-invasive estimate of myocardial preservation. The results of R wave scores and global ejection fraction measured by radionuclide scanning are given in Table 7. Again, little difference was noted between treatment and control groups either in the early entry or late entry patients. Rather anomalously, the numbers here suggest better R wave preservation in the late entry group.

Table 6. Preliminary follow-up data for the 149 patients in the APSAC study

	Median time 10.5		Months	
	Early		Late	
	Treatment	Control	Treatment	Control
Entered	38	38	37	36
Discharged	38	35	35	34
Renewed	28	32	29	23
Deaths during f/u	2	1	4	6
Lost to f/u	3	2	2	2

Table 7. Preliminary R wave score and ejection fraction data at follow-up in the early- and late-entry groups

	Early		Late	
	Treatment	Control	Treatment	Control
R-wave score	32	33	28	17
Ejection fraction	38	45	43	40

Conclusion

We began our pragmatic study of this interesting compound with the premise that, given intravenously, APSAC provides high thrombolytic activity at sites of recent thrombus. From our study of 149 patients with suspected acute myocardial infarction we endorse the fact that APSAC is simple to give and relatively safe. There were certainly no early haemodynamic disadvantages to its administration – and there were strong hints from indirect evidence that reperfusion occurred leading to myocardial salvage (Tables 1, 2, and 4).

The advantages of using APSAC in acute coronary occlusion arise from its time-course of action, its safety, and its simplicity of use. Its satisfactory time-activity curve allows thrombolytic activity to be achieved rapidly but to be prolonged for several hours beyond its administration as a single intravenous bolus. The need for an intravenous infusion is precluded. This benefit, coupled with the fact that no adverse haemodynamic effects were seen following the administration of APSAC, may enable the earliest possible administration of thrombolytic therapy in patients with evolving infarction, outside hospital by the primary care physician or paramedic.

In spite of its fibrin-specificity we found APSAC to have a modest systemic effect. This was observed not only in the bruising and occasional bleeding, but also in that the level of plasma fibrinogen in patients after infarction was lower in the treated than in the control group. (Data still under analysis.) In a separate study of more than 750 patients we have examined the rise of plasma fibrinogen following acute myocardial infarction. In our laboratory a rise in all infarct patients is seen above the normal range (2–4) to an average level of 7 g/l. Patients receiving APSAC appear to have fibrinogen levels at around 2 g/l or below, somewhere between 50 and 75% of the normal level. But this may not be a disadvantage; a modest systemic effect may in practice have a beneficial action in opposing arterial reocclusion (10), a phenomenon that threatens when treatment with the alternative short-acting agent TPA is discontinued.

To summarise, anisoylated-plasminogen-streptokinase-activator complex, APSAC, is an effective compound for intravenous thrombolytic therapy in acute coronary occlusion. Patients with developing acute myocardial infarction are most likely to benefit if they receive treatment within the first 2½ hours after the onset of major symptoms. This agent may be especially useful in hospitals without invasive facilities, and may be appropriate for use before hospital admission.

References

1. Been M, de Bono DP, Boulton FE (1984) Acute coronary thrombolysis with a single intracoronary injection of BRL 26921. (Abstr) Br Heart J 51:679
2. Been M, de Bono DP, Muir AL, Boulton FE, Hillis WS, Hornung R (1985) Coronary thrombolysis with intravenous anisoylated plasminogen streptokinase complex BRL 26921. Br Heart J 53:253–259
3. Dupe RJ, English PD, Smith RAG, Green J (1984) Acyl-enzymes as thrombolytic agents in dog models of venous thrombosis and pulmonary embolism. Thromb Haemost 51:248–283
4. Fears R, Green J, Smith RAG, Walker P (1985) Induction of a sustained fibrinolytic response by BRL 26921 in vitro. Thromb Res 38:251–260
5. Hoffman JJML, Van Rey FJW, Bonnier JJRM (1985) Systemic effects of BRL 26921 during thrombolytic treatment of acute myocardial infarction. Thromb Res 37:567–572
6. Kasper W, Erbel R, Meinertz T et al. (1984) Intracoronary thrombolysis with an acylated streptokinase-plasminogen activator (BRL 26921) in patients with acute myocardial infarction. J Am Coll Cardiol 4:357–363
7. Marder VJ, Rothbard RL, Fitzpatrick PG, Francis CW, Smith EK, Rogal GL (1984) Dose-response study of intravenous acylated streptokinase-plasminogen complex (BRL 26921) in coronary artery thrombosis. Circulation 70 (Suppl II):29
8. Matsuo O, Collen D, Verstraete M (1981) On the fibrinolytic and thrombolytic properties of active-site p anisoylated-streptokinase-plasminogen-complex (BRL 26921). Thromb Res 24:347–358
9. Norris RM, Brandt PWT, Caughey DE, Lee AJ, Scott PJ (1969) A new coronary prognostic index. Lancet i:274–278
10. Rothbard RL, Fitzpatrick PG, Francis CW, Caton RN, Hood WB, Marder VJ (1985) Relationship of the lytic state to successful reperfusion with standard- and low-dose intracoronary streptokinase. Circulation 71:562–570
11. Smith RAG, Dupe RJ, English PD, Green J (1981) Fibrinolysis with acyl-enzymes: a new approach to thrombolytic therapy. Nature 290:505–508
12. Walker ID, Davidson JF, Rae AP, Hutton I, Lawrie TDV (1984) Acylated streptokinase-plasminogen complex in patients with acute myocardial infarction. Thromb Haemost 51:204–206

Author's address

R. Vincent, M.D.
Cardiac Department
Royal Sussex County Hospital
Eastern Road
Brighton BN3 6QL
U.K.

31

Discussion

PASSAMANI:

Was the study not blinded? Also, you showed the overall figures; was there a greater difference in the early as opposed to late treatment groups?

VINCENT:

It was not blinded to the investigators. The patients treated early did better than those treated later.

LUBSEN:

You showed some effects on the eventual number of infarcts that were confirmed. Did you do your enzyme area under the curve calculations only for the confirmed infarcts or for the whole group?

VINCENT:

We estimated them both. The figures presented were only for those which had gone on to confirmed infarction.

JULIAN:

Can you tell us the incidence of ventricular fibrillation in the two groups?

VINCENT:

There was no difference. It was in the order of 8–10% in both groups.

SCHWERT:

You did not report any adverse haemodynamic effects. How did you measure blood pressure, because with an intra-arterial line we had a drop in systolic blood pressure of about 60 mm of mercury in the first 15 min. I would consider that as a marked haemodynamic effect.

VINCENT:

Yes, I accept that. We did not use intra-arterial monitoring. The patients received their bolus dose in the Accident and Emergency Unit with conventional blood pressure recording. So that the observation that it did not produce any early haemodynamic effects was based on the appearance of the patient and the pulse. We were aware that a marked drop in blood pressure has been reported when the agent is given intravenously in some people. It was partly for this reason that we used an infusion time of 4 min in the initial administration of the drug.

Question:

Why do you think that APSAC prevents reocclusion?

VINCENT:

We have no evidence to this effect. We are aware that thrombolytic activity continues for several hours after the initial infusion. This may be a useful effect, but we have not examined it ourselves as we do not have the facilities.

Question:

There is some evidence that after APSAC there is hardly any reocclusion in the first six days. Now, one cannot expect the fibrolytical activity to persist for so long.

VINCENT:

Yes, I agree. This poses a complicated problem.

Question:

When BRL was introduced one of the major disadvantages was fever. Did you ever have any patient with fever?

VINCENT:

We had no unexpected fevers. Plainly in the course of acute myocardial infarction some patients develop small degrees of fever. But there was nothing which appeared remarkably or differently related to those receiving APSAC.

Antifibrin-urokinase complex

C. Bode, M. S. Runge, G. R. Matsueda, and E. Haber

Boston (U.S.A.)

Tissue plasminogen activator (t-PA) and pro-urokinase have been compared favourably to streptokinase and urokinase on account of localization of fibrinolytic activity to the site of the clot. It is also clear that there is still room for improvement. The strategy we utilize to increase the selectivity of urokinase for fibrin is to couple the enzyme to an agent that targets it to fibrin, namely a fibrin specific monoclonal antibody.

Fibrinogen is a symmetrical macromolecule comprised of two identical subunits, each composed of three polypeptide chains termed alpha, beta, and gamma chains. Fibrinogen is converted to fibrin monomer by the cleavage of two small peptides, fibrinopeptide A and fibrinopeptide B from the alpha and beta chains. The fact that there is 98% identity in the primary structures of fibrin and fibrinogen has made it very difficult in the past to raise antibodies that differentiated between these two molecules.

Figure 1 shows a magnification of the center portion of the fibrin monomer molecule. Thrombin has now cleaved the alpha and beta chains and two new amino termini are revealed. We centered our attention on the amino terminus of the beta chain, the sequence of which is spelled out in Fig. 2. A peptide corresponding to this epitope was synthesized. It consisted of the seven amino terminal residues of the beta chain of human fibrin plus a cysteine residue that allowed covalent binding through

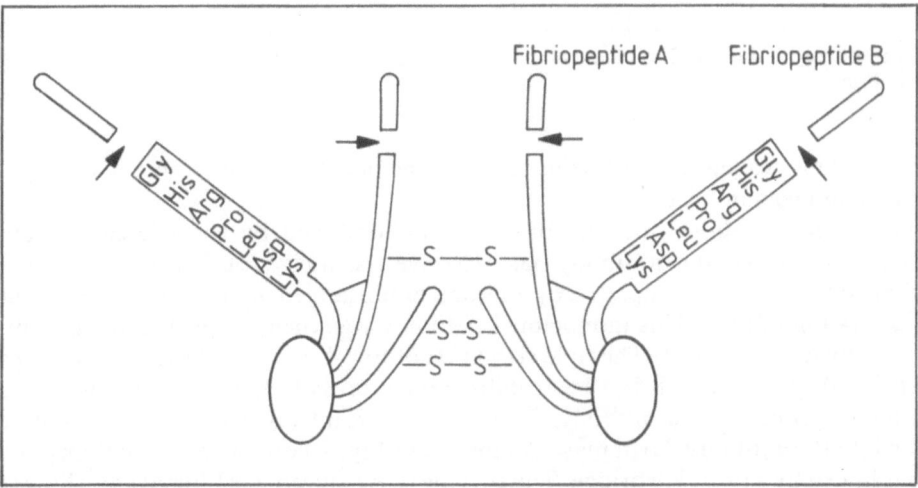

Fig. 1. Thrombin cleavage of fibrinopeptide B from fibrinogen exposes a new fibrin-specific site, B-beta 15-22

35

| Gly-His-Arg-Pro-Leu-Asp-Lys | -Cys-MBS-KLH |

Fig. 2. A synthetic peptide corresponding to the B-beta 15-22 epitope was linked to a carrier protein and served as an immunogen in mice

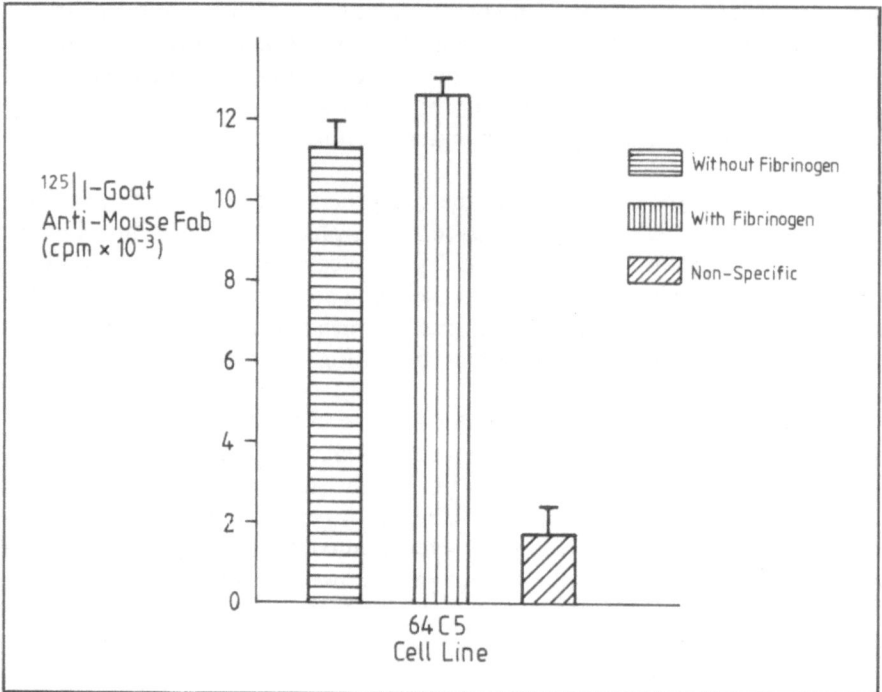

Fig. 3. Specificity of the anti-fibrin monoclonal antibody: fibrinogen does not interfere with its binding to fibrin

a cross-linking reagent to the carrier protein. The peptide-carrier complex was used as an immunogen in mice.

A monoclonal antibody specific for fibrin was obtained by somatic cell fusion. Figure 3 shows that this antibody has exclusive specificity for fibrin, because the binding to fibrin was not impaired by addition of fibrinogen in physiological concentrations (4 mg/ml) (4). This monoclonal antibody was then coupled to the plasminogen activator urokinase. The right hand side of Fig. 4 shows that the antibody was reacted with SPDP, which is a heterobifunctional cross-linking reagent and reacts with amino groups on the antibody. By this means, we introduced a reactive disulfide group into the antibody. Urokinase, on the left of Fig. 4, consists of two polypeptide chains linked by a disulfide bridge. The enzyme was reduced, gel filtered and allowed to react with the derivatized antibody, resulting in the formation of an intermolecular disulfide bridge (3).

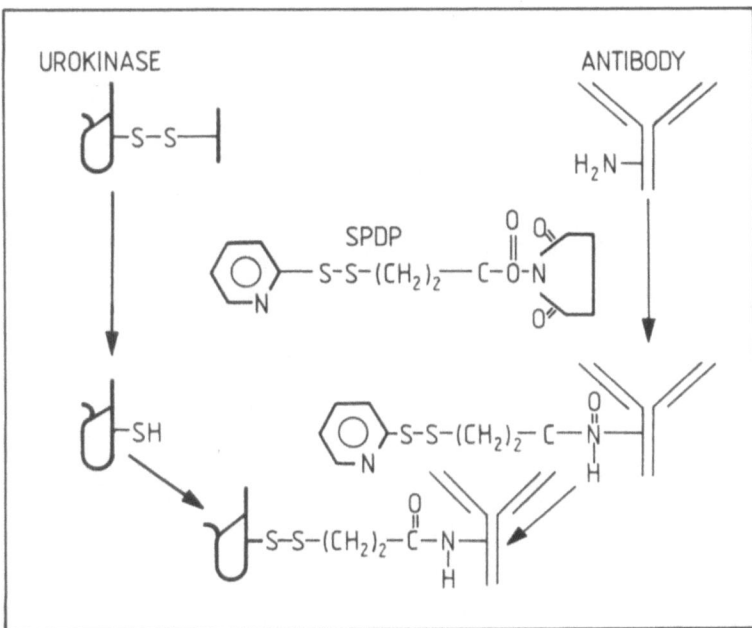

Fig. 4. Coupling reaction of antifibrin antibody and urokinase

In order to characterize the conjugate, the reaction mixture was applied to a calibrated Sephacryl S-300 column. Three protein peaks were obtained, one in the void volume of the column, the second at about 180 KD and the third at about 30 KD. Aliquots from each peak were subjected to SDS polyacrylamide gel electrophoresis and subsequent autoradiography. Urokinase had been radioactively labelled prior to coupling.

Figure 5 gives us the following information:

1. Covalent linkage of urokinase and antibody had indeed taken place since radioactivity for urokinase is now associated with a 180 KD molecule, which corresponds well to a complex of urokinase of molecular weight 30 and an antibody of 150 KD.

2. The first peak on this elution curve contains high molecular weight aggregates, peak two a conjugate of one urokinase and one antibody molecule and peak three unbound urokinase.

To fully purify the conjugate for functional studies we used a two-step affinity procedure (Fig. 6). The components in the reaction mixture are urokinase and antibody and the desired conjugate. First, molecules containing a urokinase catalytic site were bound to a Sepharose column to which Benzamidine, a urokinase inhibitor was linked. At this step antibody not linked to urokinase is removed in the wash and acid elution recovers a mixture of antibody-urokinase conjugate and uncoupled urokinase. This mixture is then applied to a column substituted with the heptapeptide against which the antibody was raised. At this point the urokinase not linked to the antibody is removed in the wash and acid elution yields the antibody-urokinase conjugate (2).

37

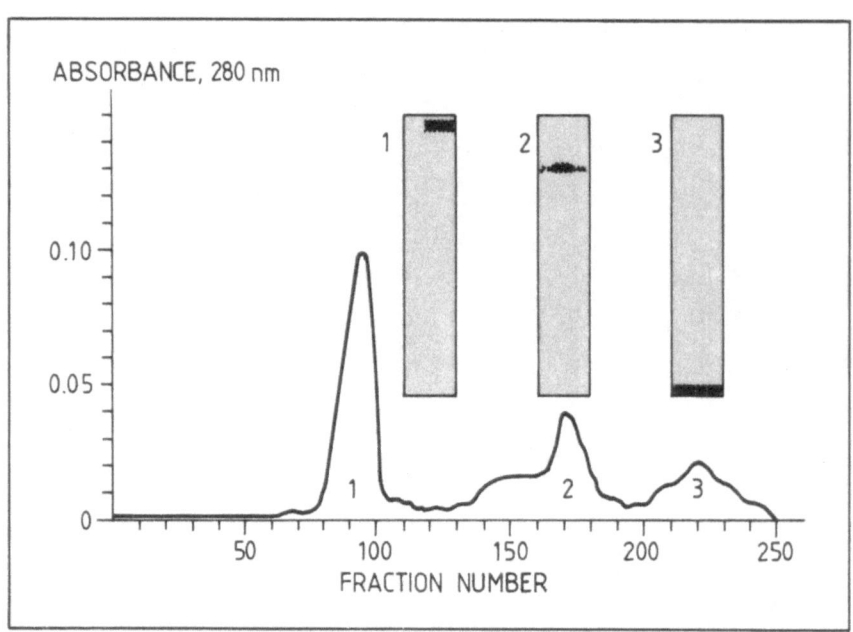

Fig. 5. Molecular characterization of the urokinase-antifibrin complex

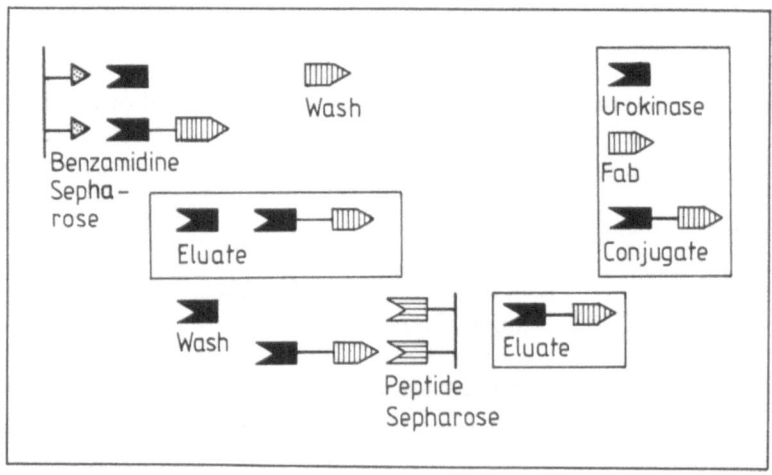

Fig. 6. Double affinity purification of urokinase-antifibrin complexes from the reaction mixture

The assay which we used to evaluate the functional activity of these compounds utilized iodine 125 labelled fibrin-monomer linked to Sepharose. The fibrin monomers were incubated with different amounts of activator (either antibody bound urokinase or urokinase alone) (Fig. 7). We also had a control conjugate consisting of an antibody of irrelevant specificity coupled to urokinase. The test plasminogen activator is added together with plasminogen and the release of labelled peptides is measured.

38

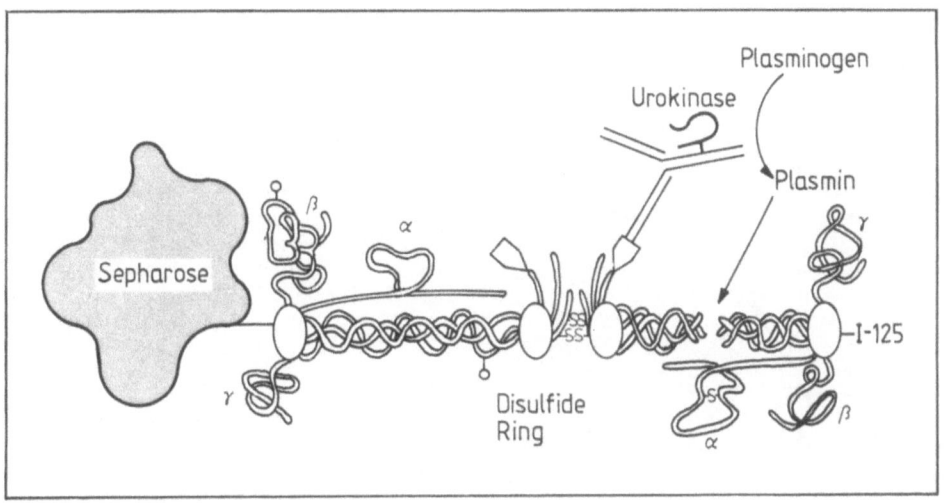

Fig. 7. Fibrin-Sepharose assay for quantitative assessment of fibrinolytic potency

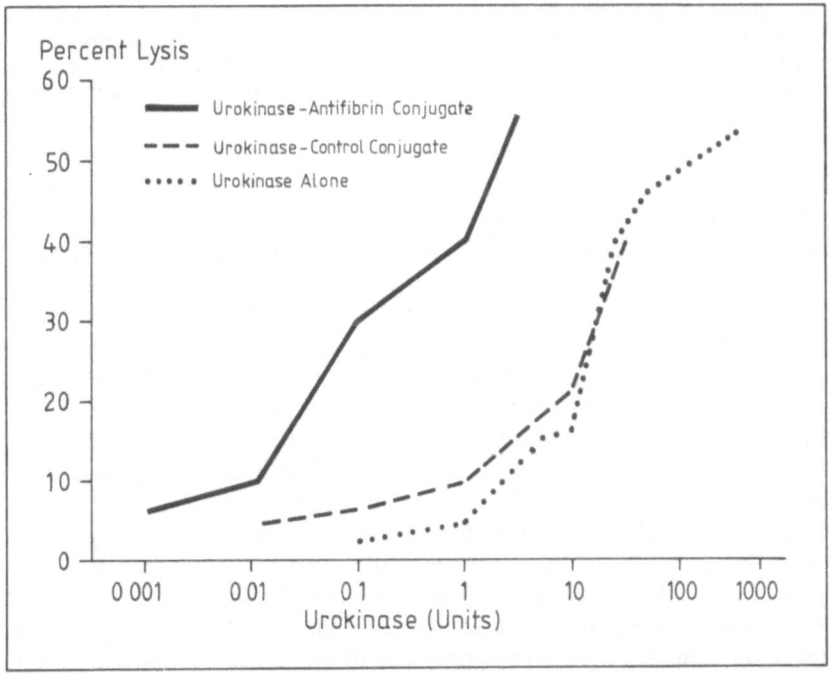

Fig. 8. Comparison of fibrinolysis achieved at different concentrations of urokinase-antifibrin complex (far left), urokinase-control-conjugate and uncoupled urokinase (right). Urokinase-antifibrin complex is 100 times more effective than the controls. Reproduced from Bode C. et al. (1985) Science 229:765–769, with permission (1). Copyright 1985 by the American Association for the Advancement of Science

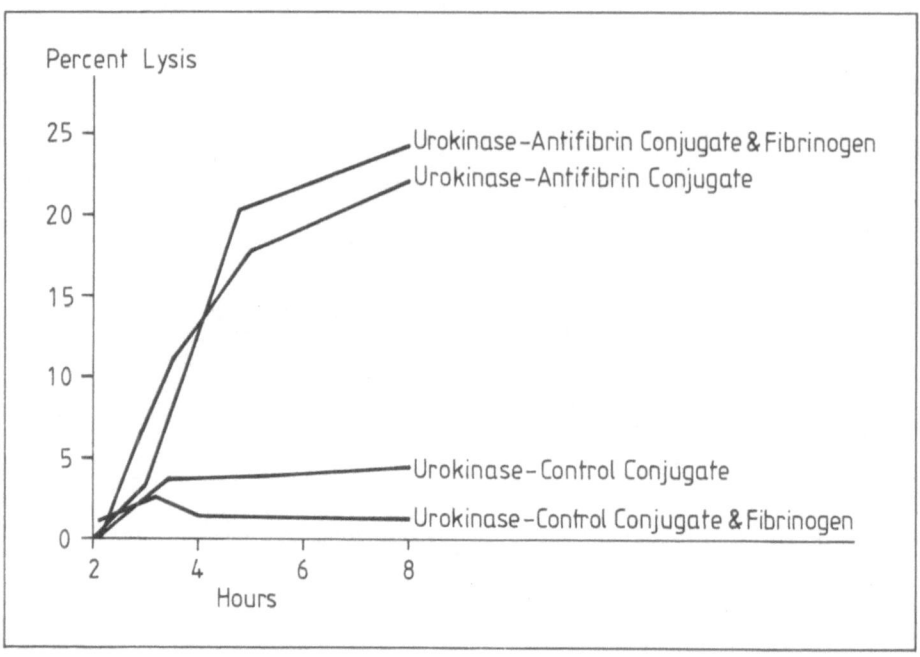

Fig. 9. Fibrinolysis achieved over time in the presence and absence of fibrinogen. The enhancement of fibrinolysis by the urokinase-antifibrin complex is independent of the presence of fibrinogen, highlighting the fibrin specificity of the complex. Reproduced from Bode C. et al. (1985) Science 229:765–769, with permission (1). Copyright 1985 by the American Association for the Advancement of Science

Percent lysis is defined as the fraction of radioactivity released from the resin to total radioactivity initially present on the resin.

Figure 8 shows the results of this assay. Percent lysis is plotted against the units of urokinase that we used. The three curves represent the urokinase antifibrin conjugate, urokinase alone, and the control conjugate described above. We must stress that this is a log scale and that the effect we can achieve with ten units of urokinase can be achieved with only 0.1 unit of antifibrin urokinase conjugate. There is thus about a 100-fold difference in efficacy of fibrin monomer lysis. On the other hand, urokinase alone and the control conjugate did not differ significantly from each other. In order to obtain kinetic information the antifibrin conjugate and the control conjugate were continuously circulated over a small column containing 125 iodine labelled fibrin Sepharose. The circulating fluid contained buffer, plasminogen and 0.25 U urokinase/100 µl linked to either the antifibrin antibody or the control antibody. The results are presented in Fig. 9. Urokinase control conjugate did not elicit any lysis, whereas considerable lysis was achieved by the antifibrin conjugate. The same experiment was then repeated in the presence of physiological concentrations of fibrinogen (3.5 mg/ml). The enhancement of fibrinolysis achieved with the urokinase antifibrin conjugate was not impaired by the presence of fibrinogen (Fig. 9), again highlighting the fibrin specificity of this new agent (1).

To conclude, in keeping with the title of this volume we will first summarize the facts. We were able to attach urokinase to a targeting device to fibrin, while retaining en-

40

zyme activity. The hybrid molecule enhances lysis of fibrin 100-fold as compared to uncoupled urokinase. Thirdly, and importantly, physiological concentrations of fibrinogen do not interfere with the enhancement of fibrinolysis.

We now turn to our hopes for the future. Fibrin-specific antibodies, which bind five times as avidly to fibrin as the antibody used in this study are now available in our laboratory. We plan to use such antibodies in the construction of new conjugates. Evidence exists that the urokinase antifibrin complex binds more tightly to fibrin than does t-PA. Conjugates of t-PA or pro-urokinase with a fibrin-specific antibody might thus result in higher affinity for fibrin, while still retaining the desirable inactivity of these agents in the circulation. And thirdly, other epitopes on fibrin or on platelets need to be explored as targets for monoclonal antibodies carrying clot dissolving agents.

References

1. Bode C, Matsueda GR, Hui KY, Haber E (1985) Antibody directed urokinase: a specific fibrinolytic agent. Science 229:765–767
2. Bode C, Runge MS, Matsueda GR, Haber E (In preparation)
3. Carlsson J, Drevin H, Axen R (1978) Protein thiolation and reversible protein-protein conjugation. Biochem J 173:723–737
4. Hui KY, Haber E, Matsueda GR (1983) Monoclonal antibodies to a synthetic fibrin-like peptide bind to human fibrin but not fibrinogen. Science 222:1129–1131

Authors' address:

Christoph Bode, M.D.
Ruprecht-Karls-Universität
Medizinische Klinik
Abteilung Innere Medizin III
Bergheimer Straße 58
6900 Heidelberg 1
West Germany

Discussion

Question:

Dr. Bode, have your already done some animal experiments in vivo with the conjugated urokinase?

BODE:

The only in vivo experiments that have been performed so far are preliminary imaging studies with the antifibrin antibody. The antibody is indeed able to visualize clots in coronary arteries, which makes us hopeful that we can achieve lysis. No conjugate has been injected into any animal so far.

Question:

Do you have any assurance that the complex does not dissociate in vivo?

BODE:

We have performed preliminary studies with plasma as the medium, which were carried out at 37 degrees during which the complex remained fairly stable. I cannot yet tell whether it will work in vivo.

Question:

Is rapid clearance of the complex not a problem?

BODE:

Clearance of this complex can really be tailored to the needs that occur because you can take either the whole antibody or fractions of the antibody. You might eventually also be able to just take fractions of the enzyme. The ultimate aim is naturally to produce this agent with just an antibody combining site and an active enzyme site by recombinant techniques.

GISSI – A randomized trial with intravenous streptokinase in acute myocardial infarction. Preliminary results

F. Rovelli and F. Mauri

On behalf of the Gruppo Italiano per lo Studio della Streptochinasi nell' Infarcto Miocardico
Divisione Cardiologica, Ospedale Niguarda, Milan (Italy)

In 1983 the first meeting of Italian cardiologists took place in Milan to draw up the protocol for the study of streptokinase in myocardial infarction, the GISSI trial. The scientific committee, having obtained all the information available at that time (1–3, 5–14, 16), decided to test the effects of brief duration, intravenous administration of streptokinase on in-hospital mortality, medium term mortality, six and twelve months mortality, and type and frequency of cardiac morbidity within six months of treatment. As the in-hospital mortality for acute myocardial infarction previously estimated in Italy by a specific enquiry ranged between 12 and 15%, we needed to recruit about 11000 patients in order to demonstrate a statistically significant reduction of 20%. This reduction was considered the main clinical endpoint. In order to ensure maximum cooperation from the coronary care units (CCU) active at that time in Italy, the protocol had to be very simple. The study was planned following a controlled multicentre open level design with central randomization (4–15). The co-operating centres had to comply with only very few operative steps.

Methods

After admission to CCU all the patients were screened for eligibility criteria. Signs and symptoms suggestive of acute myocardial infarction, i.e. chest pain lasting more than 20 min, and ST-segment deviation of 1 mm or more in any limb lead or 2 mm or more in any precordial lead. Admission to CCU within twelve hours from onset of symptoms was the second condition, and the third was no clear contraindication to streptokinase treatment.

Ineligible patients had to be registered in a reject log containing their essential information which will be evaluated separately. Figure 1 summarizes the major operative steps of the protocol. The pre-treatment measurements consisted of the twelve standard lead ECG and blood sampling for streptokinase (SK). Patients were then randomized by a telephone call to the coordinating centre where an around-the-clock secretariat service was available to consult a computer-generated list for blocks and stratification by hospital. The patients allocated to the treatment group received 1 500 000 IU of SK in 60 min. The other patients received the routine diagnostic and therapeutic measures normally taken in each hospital. The only difference between the two groups was the lack of thrombolytic treatment for the control group. All co-operating centres were firmly recommended to avoid different therapeutic approaches for treated and untreated patients. A check was made to verify this condition. At transfer from the CCU and again at discharge from hospital, the clinician had to complete forms concerning the main prognostic factors, the most important

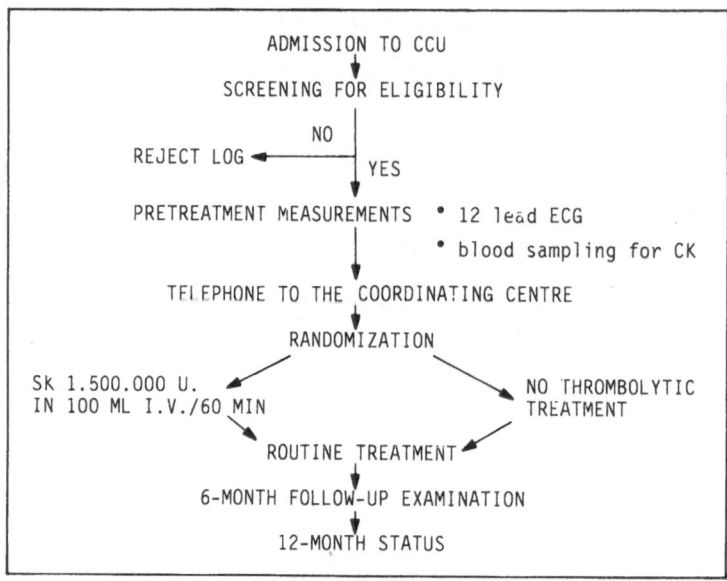

```
                    ADMISSION  TO  CCU
                            ↓
                 SCREENING  FOR  ELIGIBILITY

                          NO
         REJECT LOG ◄─────────────
                          ┃    YES

           PRETREATMENT  MEASUREMENTS    •  12 lead ECG
                          ┃              •  blood sampling for CK
                          ↓
          TELEPHONE  TO  THE  COORDINATING  CENTRE
                          ↓
                    RANDOMIZATION

    SK 1.500.000 U.   ◄                    ►  NO THROMBOLYTIC
    IN 100 ML I.V./60 MIN                     TREATMENT
                    ►  ROUTINE  TREATMENT  ◄
                          ↓
             6-MONTH  FOLLOW-UP  EXAMINATION
                          ↓
                   12-MONTH  STATUS
```

Fig. 1. Major operative steps of the protocol.

clinical events, and the basic treatment given. These two forms were reviewed at the coordinating centre by two other clinicians, who, when necessary, could ask for the clarification of a dubious answer. All the data were analyzed on an intention to treat principle. Differences concerning the prevalence of mortality were also evaluated on the basis of time elapsed from onset of symptoms to randomization. Complementary protocols dealing with some specific problem – ECG evolution, serum enzyme levels, arrhythmias, coronary anatomy, and regional contractility – were also drawn up and executed by the cooperating centres. The data of the few patients studied under these protocols will shortly be available. A total of 11 806 patients were randomized by 176 participating CCUs throughout Italy over a period of 17 months from January 1984 to July 1985. This means that about 40% of all patients hospitalized for myocardial infarction were randomized. Perfect balance was achieved between the two halves for the most important angiographic and clinical features and therapeutic procedures.

Results

The results presented in Table 1 concern 10 732 patients analyzed so far. Shortly the correctly reviewed forms of all patients will be available and we shall be able to analyze all the cases. Table 1 lists the overall in-hospital mortality in relation to treatment. The difference between the two groups in favour of streptokinase is statistically significant with a reduction of 15% in mortality in the SK group. It is noteworthy that the mortality expected in the protocol, which was 12%, is very close to that actually observed (11.6%).

44

Table 1. Mortality by treatment

% (No. deaths/No. pts)			
SK	C	Overall	p
10.7	12.5	11.6	0.006
(576/5360)	(670/5372)	(1246/10732)	

Table 2. Mortality by hours from onset of symptoms

	% (No. deaths/No. pts)			
	SK	C	Overall	p
≤3	9.3	11.9	10.6	0.001
	(285/3054)	(370/3115)	(655/6169)	
>3–6	11.7	12.9	12.3	n.s.
	(175/1496)	(181/1399)	(356/2895)	
>6–9	13.3	14.4	13.8	n.s.
	(74/558)	(83/578)	(157/1136)	
>9–12	17.1	12.9	14.9	n.s.
	(42/245)	(35/272)	(77/517)	

Table 2 shows the mortality data subdivided by time elapsed between the onset of symptoms and the randomization. Percentage mortality reduction is related to time from the onset of chest pain with a statistically significant reduction in patients treated within 3 h (about 20%). The positive trend is present until 9 h with different reductions in mortality of about 10% between 3 h and 6 h and of about 7% between 6 h and 9 h. The trend reverses afterwards but without a definite negative effect. The first and second groups are sufficiently larger to allow a good estimate of the actual difference in mortality, while the other groups are too small to draw any conclusions. The mortality reduction reaches 47% in patients randomized to streptokinase within the first hour from onset of symptoms and the difference is highly significant from a statistical point of view. The following analyses not specifically planned in the original protocol give some indication of the groups of patients in whom SK treatment appears to have different effects. With a larger number of patients stratification can be done *a posteriori* to reliably assess the effect of SK in various subgroups, according to age, sex, location, and severity of infarction, and other associated features. However, even when differences between groups have been found to be statistically significant, the results must nevertheless be interpreted merely as strongly suggestive hypotheses and cannot necessarily be translated into definite conclusions.

Streptokinase appears to be more effective in reducing mortality in patients under 65 years of age. The figures were 7.3 for untreated patients and 5.6 for SK patients. A difference of 23%, however, as a positive trend is present in patients over 65 years of age (Table 3). Patients with previous myocardial infarction do not seem to benefit by treatment with SK, while those with the first episode have a mortality reduction

Table 3. Mortality by age

	% (No. deaths/No. pts)			
	SK	C	Overall	p
≤65	5.6 (196/3498)	7.3 (254/3457)	6.5 (450/6955)	0.03
66–75	16.8 (220/1313)	17.3 (230/1331)	17.0 (450/2644)	n.s.
≥75	29.0 (159/548)	32.1 (186/580)	30.6 (345/1128)	n.s.

Table 4. Mortality by previous infarcts

	% (No. deaths/No. pts)			
	SK	C	Overall	p
No	9.7 (434/4474)	12.0 (541/4527)	12.8 (975/9001)	0.007
Yes	16.2 (139/859)	15.5 (126/814)	15.8 (265/1673)	n.s.

Table 5. Mortality by sex

	% (No. deaths/No. pts)			
	SK	C	Overall	p
M	8.7 (371/4289)	10.2 (438/4301)	9.4 (809/8590)	0.01
F	19.1 (204/1070)	21.7 (232/1070)	20.4 (436/2140)	n.s.

of about 19% (Table 4). The effects on males and females seem to be the same, although statistical significance emerges only for the group of males which is large and not for the group of females which is smaller. From an epidemiological point of view, it is interesting to note that the overall mortality of females is twice that of males (Table 5).

Concerning the influence of site of infarction, anterior and multiple site infarctions appear to benefit more than the others with a 20% reduction of mortality in anterior infarction and a 30% reduction in multiple location (Table 6).

The possibility of assessing the benefit risks profile of SK in such a large control trial must be mentioned. Table 7 shows the distribution of the main side effects of the drug. In contrast with what most clinicians initially expected, routine administration of SK does not produce alarming events. Major bleeding amounted to only 0.3%,

Table 6. Mortality by site of infarction

	% (No. deaths/No. pts)			
	SK	C	Overall	p
Inferior	6.9 (125/1819)	6.6 (122/1848)	6.7 (247/3867)	n.s.
Anterior	14.5 (254/1752)	18.1 (333/1844)	16.3 (587/3596)	0.004
Lateral	9.5 (27/284)	6.3 (14/224)	8.1 (41/508)	n.s.
Multiple location	9.9 (94/951)	14.4 (129/898)	12.1 (223/1849)	0.0003
No Q-waves	19.9 (42/211)	16.7 (36/215)	18.3 (78/426)	n.s.
Other	9.7 (31/321)	9.6 (31/322)	9.6 (62/643)	n.s.

Table 7. Side effects in 5,360 patients randomized to SK

	No.	%
Major bleeding	19	0.3
Minor bleeding	198	3.7
Allergic reaction	131	2.4
Hypotension	159	3.0
Anaphyilactic shock	6	0.1
Fever and shiver	58	1.1

Table 8. Non-fatal cardiac events (10,732 patients)

	SK	C
Reinfarction	180	92
Pericarditis	325	565
Left ventricular failure	583	671
Post-infarction angina	812	772
Pulmonary and systemic thromboembolism	24	50

probably because SK treatment was not followed by anticoagulant in the large majority of cases. Many patients were treated with antiplatelet drugs. We also have a low incidence of allergic reactions.

With regard to the major non-fatal cardiac events, the following findings are worthy of note (Table 8). There is a higher incidence of reinfarction in patients treated with SK. This can probably be attributed to early recanalization and subsequent reocclusion. There is also a lower incidence of pericarditis in treated patients that could be attributed to the limitation of the infarct size by SK. Even the lower incidence of pulmonary and systemic thromboembolism could be attributed to the pharmacological action of streptokinase.

In conclusion, the GISSI study indicates an overall benefit of streptokinase on in-hospital mortality, especially for patients treated within three hours from onset of symptoms without previous myocardial infarction, and with selected location. Naturally, we have to await the 6 and 12 months follow-up findings to see whether the beneficial effects persist in relation to long-term survival.

References

1. Braunwald E (1985) The aggressive treatment of acute myocardial infarction. Circulation 71:1087–1092
2. Intracoronary thrombolysis (Editorial) (1983) Lancet ii:606
3. Kennedy JK, Titchie JL, Davis KB, Fritz JK (1983) Western Washington randomized trial of intracoronary streptokinase in acute myocardial infarction. N Engl J Med 309:1477–1482
4. Protocol of ISIS 2 (International Studies of Infarct Survival) (1985) Radcliffe Infirmary, Oxford
5. Simoons ML, van der Brand M, De Zwaan C et al (1985) Improved survival after early thrombolysis in acute myocardial infarction. A randomised trial by the Interuniversity Cardiology Institute in the Netherlands. Lancet ii:578–581
6. Spann JF, Sherry S (1984) Coronary thrombolysis for evolving myocardial infarction. Drugs 28:465–483
7. Stampfer MJ, Goldhaber SZ, Yusuf S, Peto R, Hennekens CH (1982) Effect of intravenous streptokinase on acute myocardial infarction. Pooled results from randomized trials. N Engl J Med 307:1180–1182
8. Tendera MP, Campbell WB, Tennant SN, Ray WA (1985) Factors influencing probability of reperfusion with intracoronary ostial infusion of thrombolytic agent in patients with acute myocardial infarction. Circulation 71:124–128
9. The ISAM Study Group (1985) Intravenous Streptokinase in Acute Myocardial Infarction: preliminary results of a prospective controlled trial (ISAM). Presented at 58th Congress of the American Heart Association, Washington, Nov 10–14, 1985
10. Thrombolytic therapy in treatment. Summary of an N.I.H. consensus conference (1980). Br Med J 280:1585–1587
11. TIMI Study Group (1985) The Thrombolysis in Myocardial Infarction (TIMI) trial. Phase I findings. N Engl J Med 312:932–936
12. Verstraete M (1985) Even if the efficacy of intracoronary thrombolysis is proven, this approach is a death issue in terms of public health. In: Davidson JF, Donati MB, Cocchieri S (eds) Progress in Fibrinolysis, Vol VII. Churchill Livingstone, Edinburgh, pp 25–29
13. Verstraete M (1985) Intravenous administration of a thrombolytic agent is the only realistic therapeutic approach in evolving myocardial infarction. Eur Heart J 6:586–593
14. Verstraete M, Bernard R, Bory M et al (1985) Randomised trial of intravenous recombinant tissue-type plasminogen activator versus intravenous streptokinase in acute myocardial infarction. Lancet i:842–847
15. Yusuf S, Collins R, Peto R (1984) Why do we need some large, simple randomized trials? Stat Med 3:409–420
16. Yusuf S, Collins R, Peto R et al. (1985) Intravenous and intracoronary fibrinolytic therapy in acute myocardial infarction: overview of results on mortality, reinfarction and side-effects from 33 randomized controlled trials. Eur Heart J 6:556–585

Authors' address:

Professor F. Mauri
Divisione Cardiologica
„Centro A. de Gasperis"
Ospedale Niguarda – Ca'Granda
Piazza Ospedale Maggiore, 3
20162 Milano-Niguarda
Italy

ISAM – A randomized trial
with intravenous streptokinase versus placebo

K. L. Neuhaus for the ISAM-study group

Universitäts-Klinik Göttingen (West Germany)

The ISAM (intravenous streptokinase in acute myocardial infarction) trial is a double-blind multicentre randomized study comparing the effects of a one hour i.v. infusion of 1.5 million units of streptokinase (STK) with treatment with heparin and aspirin only. This treatment has been given to the streptokinase group as well. From 1982 to 1985, 1741 patients aged up to 75 years were included.

The trial was conducted by 38 centres, mainly German and Swiss, and during the latest phase of the studies by some Toronto clinics as well. 1573 patients were admitted to the study from West Germany and Switzerland, and 168 patients participated in Toronto: a total of 859 patients were randomly allocated to STK, with 882 in the control group. No patient was lost to follow-up. The main endpoint of the study was early and late mortality and secondary endpoints were morbidity, i.e. non-fatal critical events such as reinfarction and the limitation of infarct size as measured from ECG from CK and from ventriculography and, of course, the documentation of complications.

Figure 1 plots the overall mortality during the first 21 days of the study for the total population. There were 54 deaths in the streptokinase group compared to 63 deaths in the placebo group during the first three weeks (not statistically significant).

If we look at the cause-specific mortality by treatment group (Table 1) we can see that there is a difference of 45 cardiac deaths in the STK group versus 60 in the control group, that there is no difference in sudden and arrhythmia deaths, and that there is a death rate of 2 in every group from reinfarction. This is very low and the

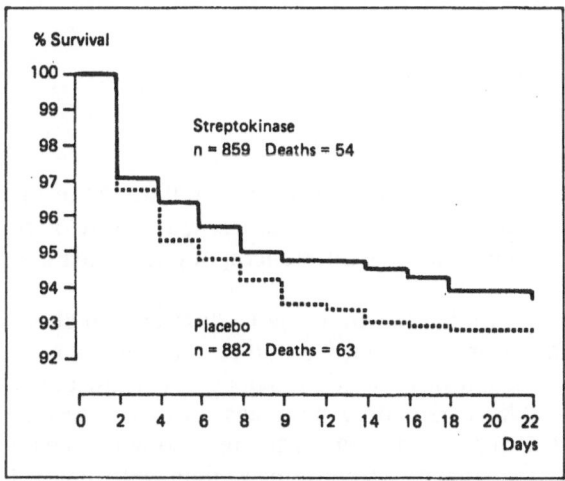

Fig. 1. 21-day-survival after acute myocardial infarction

Tabelle 1. Cause-specific mortality by treatment group. Number of patients, study medication received

	STK	Control	Relative risk
Total cardiac deaths	45	60	0.77
Sudden and arrhythmia deaths	11	12	0.94
Reinfarction	2	2	–
Cardiac failure	23	33	0.68
Rupture deaths	9	13	0.71

Table 2. 21 day mortality

	STK		Control		Relative risk
	n	%	*n*	%	
Treatment < 3 h	25/476	5.3	30/463	6.5	0.81
Cardiac mortality	49/859	5.7	62/882	7.0	0.81
Male	35/694	5.0	49/727	6.7	0.75
Age < 70 years	37/738	5.1	48/726	6.6	0.77
Hypertension	17/202	8.4	12/204	5.9	1.43
Previous MI	17/106	16.0	11/102	10.8	1.49

Table 3. 21 days non-fatal events

	STK	Control	Nominal *p*-value
Bleeding complications	5.7%	1.5%	0.0001
Early reinfarctions	2.4%	1.1%	0.04
Unstable angina	5.7%	4.0%	0.09
Early ACBS	3.3%	1.9%	0.08
VF 3–24 h after start of treatment	0.7%	1.9%	0.04
Symptomatic brady- or tachy-arrhythmias after 24 h	2.0%	3.6%	0.04

main difference is made up from patients who died from cardiac failure, 23 in the STK and 33 in the control group. Rupture deaths, a major concern, are more often seen in the control than in the STK group. All these differences, of course, are statistically not significant.

Subgroups of patients treated early, i.e. within three hours, had a difference of about 20% in total mortality, giving a relative risk of about 0.8 and cardiac mortality at the same relative risk; male patients fared a little better than females and those under 70 years of age fared better than the elderly patients. An increased risk was seen in hypertensive patients and in patients with previous myocardial infarction (MI) who had a higher risk when they were treated with streptokinase than with control (Table 2).

Table 4. Side effects during infusion of study medication

	Number of patients	
	STK	Control
Nausea, vomiting	83*	45
Hypotension	89*	26
Bradycardia	78*	30
Rash	9	2
Rigors	3	1
At least one side-effect	185*	86

Nominal p * = < 0.0001

With regard to the non-fatal events, which were judged by an independent critical event committee (Table 3) it is of note that bleeding complications amounted to 5.7% in the STK group and only 1.5% in the control group, clearly indicating an increased bleeding risk from STK therapy. Included in these bleeding complications are four intracranial bleedings, two of which were fatal, and no intracranial bleeding in the control group. The early reinfarction rate was slightly higher in the STK than in the control group, with the same applying to unstable angina.

Table 4 lists the side effects experienced during the infusion. There was a significantly higher incidence in the STK group than in the control group.

Turning to the problem of limitation of infarct size by early fibrinolysis, with regard to the ejection fraction which could be determined in 841 patients (i.e. half of the total population) there was an average difference of 3% between the STK and the control group in favour of the STK group, and there were no differences in the baseline comparions between these groups (Table 5). The difference in ejection fraction was

Table 5. Global and regional LV-function 3 weeks post-MI

	Total group		Treatment			
			≦3 h		>3 h	
	STK (423 pts)	Control (418 pts)	STK (268 pts)	Control (241 pts)	STK (150 pts)	Control (175 pts)
Ejection fraction (%)	56.9±0.7	53.8± 0.7***	57.0± 0.9	53.5± 1.0**	56.8± 1.1	54.3± 1.1
EF < 50%	30%	40%	44%	43%	27%	37%
Dyssynergic index						
30° RAO projection	225 ±9	266 ±10***	221 ±13**	267 ±13**	230 ±15	263 ±15
60° LAO projection	82 ±6	109 ±8**	75 ± 8	108 ±11*	91 ±10	113 ±14

+) = inferior infarction only (408 pts). * $p < 0.05$, ** $p < 0.01$, *** $p < 0.005$

Table 6. Serial CK-MB analysis (1444 pts)

	Total group		Treatment			
			≤3 h		>3 h	
	STK	Control	STK	Control	STK	Control
Peak CK-MB (U/l)	98 ± 2	93 ± 2	96 ± 3	99 ± 3	101 ± 4**	85 ± 3
Area under CK-MB-curve (U/l×h)	1684 ± 47	1842 ± 49*	1624 ± 58	1912 ± 66**	1764 ± 77	1742 ± 73
Time to peak CK-MB (h) from symptom onset	13.9 ± 0.2***	19.2 ± 0.2	13.1 ± 0.2***	18.4 ± 0.3	15.1 ± 0.3***	20.1 ± 0.3

* $p < 0.02$, ** $p < 0.001$, *** $p < 0.0001$

slightly higher in those treated earlier than 3 h after onset of symptoms and was lower in those treated late (n.s.). If we look at patients with an ejection fraction of less than 50% this depressed ventricular function is found more often in the control group than in the STK group, independent of early or late treatment.

With regard to regional ventricular function (Table 5), again measured three weeks after MI from the ventriculogram in the RAO projection, the dysynergic index which indicates the amount of hypokinetic and dyskinetic myocardium is significantly lower in the STK group. There is a reduction of about 15% in the total group and about 17% in the early treatment group, while in the late treatment group this difference in regional function is no longer statistically significant. The same was found in the LAO projection where only inferior infarctions have been evaluated (Table 5).

From the onset of symptoms to the peak CK the time was about 20 h in the control population and 13.8 in the streptokinase group. That means a significant reduction in time to peak CK, indicating a larger proportion of recanalized or reperfused patients in the STK group. There is no major difference between treatment within 3 h and after 3 h: this means that an early wash-out is seen significantly more often in the treatment than in the placebo group. CK peaking within 13 h of the onset of symptoms indicates a certain restoration of flow during the early phase of myocardial infarction; then there are 60% with a peak earlier than 13 h in the STK group and 20% assumably with sub-total occlusion in the placebo group.

With the early wash-out one would expect that the CK peak values would be greater in the streptokinase than in the control group. Table 6 lists the average values for 1444 patients. There is no major difference between peak CK for the treatment and the control groups and those treated early had even a somewhat lower peak value than the control group. With late treatment, however, there was as expected a higher peak in the streptokinase than in the control group. One can conclude from these data that infarct size has been limited at least to some extent. There is a smaller area under the CK curve in the STK than in the control group and this difference is almost entirely due to the difference in the early treatment group. Those treated late showed no difference.

The results of the study allow the conclusion that early mortality can be reduced by streptokinase given intravenously during the first hours of MI, although the total mortality in the studied population as a whole was so low that statistical significance in the reduction of mortality could not be reached. However, the study shows a significant reduction of infarct size measured from ECG, CK-MB and from the left ventricular angiogram. Nevertheless, the therapy carries a significant bleeding risk which may partly outweigh the benefit derived from it.

Author's address:
Prof. Dr. Karl-Ludwig Neuhaus
Universitäts-Klinik Göttingen
Med. Klinik Abteilung Kardiologie
Robert-Koch-Straße 40
3400 Göttingen
West Germany

Randomized trial with intracoronary streptokinase versus placebo (Western Washington)

Edited version of the lecture by
H. T. Dodge presented at the Symposium

University of Washington Medical School, Seattle (U.S.A.)

Introduction

The Western Washington Trial was initiated in July 1981 and was completed in 1983. It is an intracoronary streptokinase multicentre trial which included a total of 14 hospitals. The entry of patients was restricted to those less than 75 years of age. They were required to have an ST elevation, and to submit to coronary angiography. Over the period of the study 250 patients were randomised to receive either streptokinase treatment or control therapy.

Protocol

The protocol was as follows. The patients had immediate cardiac catheterization and the treatment outlined in Table 1. They were randomised after it was demonstrated that they had total occlusion of a coronary artery, and the randomisation occurred at approximately 4½ h after the onset of symptoms. So this was a medium study in terms of time from onset of symptoms. Those that did not have occlusion of a coronary artery were not randomised and were dropped from the study.

Table 1. Patient management

Immediate cardiac catheterization
Methyl prednisolone 1.0 g IV
LV cine-angiography – RAO or biplane
Selective coronary arteriography
Intracoronary NTG 0.2 mg
Thrombotic occlusion
  Yes → randomize
  No → removed from study

Results

A total of 250 patients entered the trial, 134 were in the streptokinase group, and 116 were in the control group. The mortality rates at 30 days and one year are set out in Table 2. With the further follow-up at one year there were relatively few deaths over and above those occurring in the first 30 days and it is worthwhile keeping this in mind when planning studies in the future. The majority of deaths will occur during the hospitalization, during the first 30 days. At one year, the mortality rate

Table 2. Mortality in the Western Washington Streptokinase trial

	n	30 day	One year
Streptokinase	134	5 (3.7%)	11 (8.2%)
Control	116	13 (11.2%)	17 (14.7%)
p for difference		p=0.02	p=0.10

Logistic regression was used to adjust for the baseline covariates ejection fraction, moribund state, location of MI and age.

This analysis shows that streptokinase patients had a significantly improved survival. p=0.03

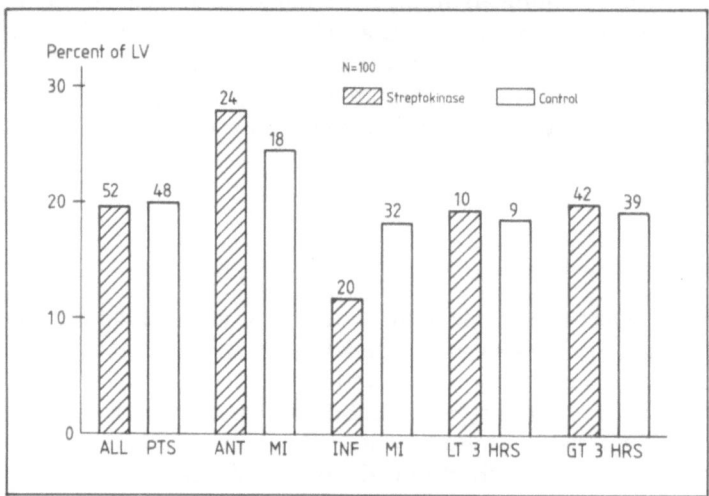

Fig. 1. Western Washington IC streptokinase trial.
Tomographic thallium infarct size

in the streptokinase treated group was 8.2% and in the control group it was 14.7%. This one year result is not statistically significant, but it transpired that in the control group there was a disproportionate number of patients with low ejection fractions and anterior infarcts. These are high risk patients for mortality and if one adjusts the results statistically to take these differences into account, then the results do become statistically significant at the p=0.03 level.

It is of interest in this study that we do have data on ventricular performance and infarct size (Fig. 1). This is radionuclide information, as determined by a tomographic thallium technique, and in spite of the differences in mortality at 30 days and at 1 year, it was not possible to demonstrate a difference in infarct size between the streptokinase treated patients and the control patients. The patients (in Fig. 1) are grouped according to the type of infarct and according to the time at which they were treated.

Again, in spite of the difference in mortality, it was not possible to demonstrate a difference in the global ejection fraction in this study (Fig. 2). This has been one of the difficult factors to explain about the study, that although there was a difference in mortality, one could not demonstrate a difference in infarct size, or in global ejec-

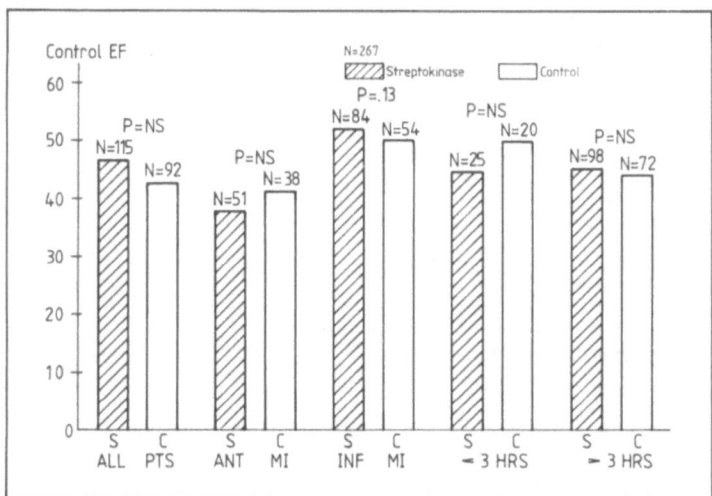

Fig. 2. 8 week ejection fraction

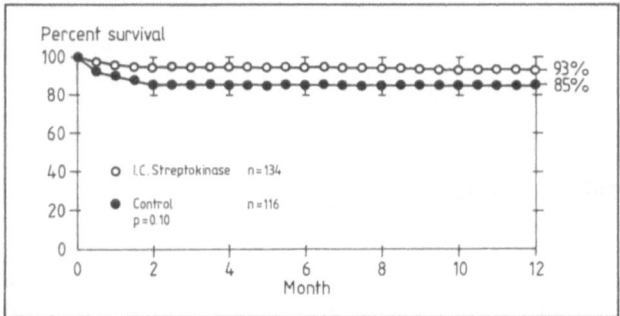

Fig. 3. Survival of streptokinase and control patients

tion fraction using these techniques. One might argue that these particular techniques may not be sensitive enough to detect the difference, or one could argue that there is some other factor important in determining mortality.

There are some other factors that we have identified as being of importance. Now, what we have done so far is to look at the results in terms of intention to treat, examining patients who received streptokinase and those who were control patients (Fig. 3). In the study as a whole, of the patients who received streptokinase, 67% achieved opening of a coronary artery. The remaining 33% did not achieve opening. If one looks instead at patients in whom the treatment was successful in opening the vessels, this picture is different: at the end of one year, the mortality rate is a little over 7% for the streptokinase treated patients and a little over 14% for the patients treated with controls.

In Fig. 4 the data are presented in terms of patients who did or did not receive successful reperfusion. In the study as a whole patients who reperfused had a one year mortality of 2.5%. There was very low mortality in the group in which the treatment was successful. Those with partial reperfusion had a mortality over 23% over one

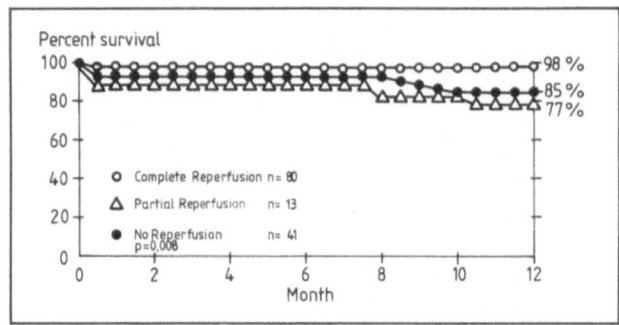

Fig. 4. Survival of treated patients by status of reperfusion

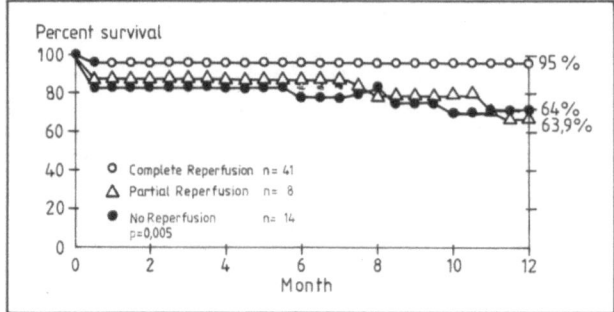

Fig. 5. Survival of patients with anterior MI by status of reperfusion

year and in those that had no reperfusion there was a mortality of 15%. This is a very striking difference. Thus, whether or not reperfusion is successful becomes another predictor of mortality in the following thrombolytic therapy.

Now this difference becomes even more striking if one looks at the types of infarcts. Figure 5 refers to patients with anterior myocardial infarcts. In those who achieved reperfusion the one year mortality was about 5%. In patients who had partial or no reperfusion, the one year mortality was in excess of 35%: a very striking difference in mortality depending on whether patients were reperfused or not.

The prognosis for patients with inferior myocardial infarcts who were treated with streptokinase is detailed in Table 3. None of the patients who had reperfusion died

Table 3. Prognosis in acute MI survival at 1 year

Multivariate analysis variables	F	P
Ejection fraction	20.0	< 0.0001
LAD stenosis or anterior ST elevation	4.4	< 0.05
Streptokinase	4.4	0.03

within the one year follow-up, whereas there was one death among the patients who failed to reperfuse. This points out another feature of the problem, that not all types of infarcts carry the same risk or mortality. The inferior infarct patients tend to be a low-risk group. With regard to the substantial discrepancies in mortality rates between various studies, one would like to ascertain how many of these patients had anterior infarcts and how many had inferior infarcts. One might even ask how one can identify patients in whom there is going to be an inferior infarction for example, and in whom it will be very difficult to demonstrate an improvement in survival, because the survival rate is so good to start with.

Summary

We have looked at several various variables as predictors of mortality and have found that ejection fraction is a very good predictor. Patients with low ejection fractions are at high risk of mortality. LAD stenosis, anterior infarction, and anterior ST elevation are all predictors; whether or not the patients receive streptokinase is a predictor of survival, and whether or not the vessel is open following streptokinase administration is also a predictor.
Multivariate analysis identified global ejection fraction and the size of infarct stenosis as being the most important baseline variables related to prognosis. It also identified streptokinase treatment as being a predictor of survival.

Conclusion

These then are the results of the Western Washington Trial, and we have done some other more sophisticated analyses of ventricular performance which also help to identify some of the patients at risk, but by and large these studies are positive in demonstrating survival. One of the unanswered questions is the basis for this, inasmuch as we were not able in these studies to identify differences in infarct size nor in ventricular performance between the control and treated groups.

References available from the author

Author's address:
Professor Harold T. Dodge
University of Washington Medical School
Seattle, WA 98195
U.S.A.

Randomized trial with intracoronary streptokinase versus placebo (The Netherlands)

M. L. Simoons[1], P. W. Serruys[1], M. v/d Brand[1], F. Bar[4], C. de Zwaan[4], J. Res[2], F. W. A. Verheugt[2], X. H. Krauss[3], W. J. Remme[3], F. Vermeer[5], and J. Lubsen[5]

[1] Thoraxcenter, Erasmus University and University Hospital Dijkzigt, Rotterdam
[2] Department of Cardiology, Free University Amsterdam
[3] Department of Cardiology, Zuiderziekenhuis, Rotterdam
[4] Department of Cardiology, St. Annadal Hospital, Maastricht
[5] Data Processing Center, Thoraxcenter, Erasmus University, Rotterdam (The Netherlands)

Introduction

In 1981 we initiated a randomized trial at the Thoraxcenter in Rotterdam which was later extended to include four other hospitals cooperating in the Netherlands Interuniversity Cardiology Institute: the Zuiderziekenhuis in Rotterdam, the Free University in Amsterdam, the St. Annadal Hospital in Maastricht and the Leiden University Hospital. Since the global results of the study have been published in the Lancet (4) and in other journals (3, 5) we present a summary of the findings and discuss the clinical consequences of the trial.

Methods and design of the trial

The study included a total of 533 patients, 264 allocated to conventional treatment without angiography, and 269 allocated to thrombolytic therapy. When the trial was started 5 years ago, we were not sure what would be the optimum method of thrombolysis, so from the outset we decided what we would be willing to alter the methods for thrombolytic therapy during the course of the trial. We made two major alterations: in the last year we started with the intravenous application of streptokinase before intracoronary application, because by that time it was evident that thrombolysis could be accelerated in that way, and secondly, we gradually learnt to perform PTCA in part of the patients, either as a method to open a vessel that was not opened by thrombolytic therapy, or as a method to prevent reocclusion, which sometimes occurred after thrombolytic therapy. Angiographic patency after the procedure was 85%.

Some specific points of our study should be emphasized. First of all, we only entered patients who arrived in the coronary care unit within 4 hours after the onset of symptoms. The median time until admission in the coronary care unit was only 90 minutes. The median time until angiographic documentation of a patent artery was 200 minutes. Thus half of the patients had an open vessel slightly more than 3 hours. That is considerably faster than, for example, the Western Washington Trial where treatment was initiated on average after 4.5 hours (1). Patients were randomized and informed consent was asked only from patients allocated to thrombolytic therapy. Conventionally treated patients did not undergo acute angiography. That is another difference from the Western Washington Trial. Patients were followed up by hemo-

61

dynamic monitoring, electrocardiography, HBDH-measurements of infarct size, radionuclide angiography, coronary arteriography and left ventriculography, exercise testing and by the out patient clinic.

Clinical data and angiographic pattency

Baseline characteristics were evenly distributed between the two groups (Table 1). About a quarter of the patients had a history of previous myocardial infarction, slightly more had a history of previous angina and, at admission, 11 patients in the control group and 12 patients allocated to thrombolytic therapy were in severe heart failure or shock. These patients were not excluded.

The angiographic results are detailed in Table 2. Two methods of treatment were used: intracoronary streptokinase only, and intracoronary streptokinase preceded by intravenous streptokinase (500 000 units given over approximately 10–15 minutes). No angiography was performed in 35 patients in spite of allocation to thrombolytic therapy. Twenty of these 35 patients refused the intervention and 15 patients were ineligible for other reasons (4). It is evident from the design of the study that,

Table 1

Base line data	Controls	Thrombolysis
Number of patients	264	269
Males	224	217
History of angina	74	69
Previous maocardial infarction	60	56
Killip I or II at admission	253	257
Killip III or IV at admission	11	12

Table 2

	Control	Thrombolysis	Angiography			
			None	○–○	●–○	●–●
Streptokinase IC only	150	152	16	25	88	23
Streptokinase IV + IC	114	117	19	40	45	13
Open at first angiogram	IC 18%	IV + IC 41%				
Open end of procedure	83%	87%				

○–○: patent vessel before and after angiography.
●–○: occluded vessel, recanalised by intracoronary streptokinase.
●–●: persistent occlusion.

62

Table 3.

Clinical course	Controls	Thrombolysis	p
Deceased (14 days)	26	14	0.05
New infarction (14 days)	9	12	
Angina (discharge)	55	57	
Heart failure (discharge)	53	37	0.05
Bleeding	7	53	0.0001

although these 35 patients did not receive thrombolytic therapy, they were analysed as part of the thrombolysis group according to the "intention to treat" principle. At the first angiogram 18% of infarct related arteries were patent in patients who were not pretreated. In patients pretreated with intravenous streptokinase 41% were open. This illustrates the advantage of intravenous streptokinase. At the end of the procedure, 83% were open in patients given intracoronary streptokinase only, and 87% were open in patients in the last year who had intravenous streptokinase. There were no differences in angiographic results between the five hospitals in the study.

The clinical course in hospital can be summarized as follows (Table 3): at 14 days 26 patients had died and 9 reinfarctions occurred in the conventionally treated group, whereas 14 patients had died and 12 had a reinfarction in the thrombolysis group. Although not statistically significant, there is already a trend towards a higher number of reinfarctions in the thrombolysis group. There was no difference in angina at hospital discharge, but there was a significant, and we think clinically very important difference in heart failure: 52 patients in the conventionally treated group and only 37 patients in the group allocated to thrombolysis. Similarly, although not statistically significant, we had more cases of cardiogenic shock in the conventionally treated group than in the thrombolysis group. Bleeding was more prominent in patients allocated to thrombolysis, but did not result in major problems in this series.

Infarct size

We measured enzymated infarct size by HBDH-release with a model which takes into account the rate of disappearance of the enzyme from the blood, and which is insensitive to the rate of release (2, 5). So, in spite of a higher release in the early hours of all enzymes (including HBDH) infarct size may still be measured. A major determinant of the effect of thrombolytic therapy as recognized from the enzymatic measurements is the delay between onset of symptoms and arrival at hospital. In patients who arrived early, within 1 hour, infarct size was half of that in patients in the thrombolytic group compared with the controls, and this difference was only 25% in patients who came in between 1 and 3 hours. There was virtually no difference in infarct size between the two groups of patients who came in late, between 3 and 4 hours after the onset of symptoms.

By multivariate analysis we demonstrated that the beneficial effects of thrombolytic therapy were mainly related to the delay between onset of symptoms and hospital

Table 4. Median values of infarct size estimated by HBDH release, left ventricular ejection fraction measured by radionuclide angiography (%) and three month mortality (%) in patients allocated to conventional treatment (C) and thrombolytic therapy (T). Data are presented in four groups of patients with total ST elevation plus ST depression > or < than 1.2 mV and with delay between onset of symptoms and hospital admission from 0–2 hours and between 2 and 4 hours.

Σ ST	delay	HBDH				Three month	
		Infarct size		LVEF (%)		mortality (%)	
		C	T	C	T	C	T
≥ 1.2	0–2	1440	820	40	48	16	7
≥ 1.2	2–4	1640	1180	44	46	17	8
< 1.2	0–2	800	500	44	57	10	4
< 1.2	2–4	680	660	52	47	8	9

admission, and to the sum of ST elevation or ST depression in the ECG at admission. These two factors were predictors of the reduction of infarct size, preservation of left ventricular function and improved survival after thrombolytic therapy.

This can be illustrated when four groups of patients are compared: patients with ST-segment changes larger than 12 mm and patients with ST-segment changes of less than 12 mm, which are both subdivided into those who arrived within 2 hours, and those who arrived between 2 and 4 hours after infarction (Table 4). There was a substantial difference in enzyme release in patients with large infarcts who came in early, and a smaller difference in those with smaller infarcts who arrived early on and in those with large infarcts who arrived later. There was no difference in infarct size in patients with electrocardiographically small infarcts who arrived late.

Left ventricular function

Preservation of global left ventricular function was documented both by contrast and radionuclide angiography (3, 5). On the average, contrast angiography showed a 47% ejection fraction in the controls and a 53% ejection fraction in the treated group. In the subgroup analysis a similar pattern as for infarct size appears from the ejection fraction data. There is an 8% difference in streptokinase allocated patients versus conventionally treated patients with a large infarct who arrived early. However, streptokinase has no effect in patients who arrived later than 2 hours with a small ST elevation.

Survival

Again, similar results can be seen when we look at mortality. Overall, patients allocated to thrombolytic therapy have a 1-year survival rate of 90%, while that for

Table 5

One year follow-up	Controls	Thrombolysis	p
n	264	269	
Acute PTCA	–	46 (17%)	
Late PTCA/CABG	42 (16%)	65 (24%)	0.02
Reinfarction	14 (5%)	36 (13%)	0.001
Death	42 (16%)	26 (10%)	0.03

the control patients is 84%. These data are very similar to the Western Washington Trial (1). In three subgroups a considerable reduction in mortality occurred, but not in patients with small infarcts who arrived later than 2 hours after the onset of symptoms.

As might be expected, there was a higher incidence of reinfarction in patients allocated to thrombolytic therapy. At the follow-up, which varied from 3 to 48 months (median follow-up 1 year), there were 36 non-fatal reinfarctions in patients allocated to thrombolytic therapy and only 16 in the conventionally treated group. Reinfarction occurred mostly in patients with an inferior wall infarction at admission (4). In addition, bypass surgery for post-infarction angina was performed more frequently in patients allocated to thrombolytic therapy (Table 5). Most reinfarctions occurred within the first three months. Thus measures to prevent these reinfarctions must certainly be performed within three months and probably within the first few days of the infarct.

Conclusion

We can conclude from this large study that early intracoronary thrombolytic therapy results in 85% angiographic patency, 30% limitation of infarct size, preservation of global and regional left ventricular function and improved 1 year survival. Best results were obtained in patients with a short treatment delay and in patients with extensive myocardial ischemia (large ST elevation) at admission. The major problem that we have encountered is more frequent reinfarction, and we hope that we will find the means to overcome this problem in the future.

References

1. Kennedy JW, Ritchie JL, Davis KB, Fritz JK (1983) Western Washington randomized trial of intracoronary streptokinase in acute myocardial infarction. N Engl J Med 308:1312–1318
2. Laarse A vd, Vermeer F, Hermens WT, Willems GM, Neef K de, Simoons ML, Serruys PW, Res J, Verheugt FWA, Krauss XH, Bär F, Zwaan C de, Lubsen J (1986) Effects of early intracoronary streptokinase on infarct size estimated from cumulative enzyme release and on enzyme release rate. Am Heart J (in press)

3. Serruys PW, Simoons ML, Suryapranata H, Vermeer F, Wijns W, Brand M vd, Bär F, Zwaan C de, Krauss XH, Remme WJ, Res J, Verheugt FWA, Domburg R van, Lubsen L, Hugenholtz PG (1986) Preservation of global and regional left ventricular function after early thrombolysis in acute myocardial infarction. JACC 7:717–728
4. Simoons ML, Serruys PW, Brand M vd, Bär F, Zwaan C de, Res J, Verheugt FWA, Krauss XH, Remme WJ, Vermeer F, Lubsen J (1985) Improved survival after early thrombolysis in acute myocardial infarction. A randomized trial conducted by the Interuniversity Cardiology Institute in the Netherlands. Lancet II:578–582
5. Simoons ML, Serruys PW, Brand M vd, Res J, Verheugt FWA, Krauss XH, Remme WJ, Bär F, Zwaan C de, Laarse A vd, Vermeer F, Lubsen J (1986) Early thrombolysis in acute myocardial infarction: limitation of infarct size and improved survival. JACC 7:729–742

Authors' address:

M. L. Simoons, M.D.
Academisch Ziekenhuis
Thoraxcentrum/Cardiologie
Molewaterplein 40
3015 GD Rotterdam
The Netherlands

Randomised trial with intravenous acylated streptokinase (BRL 26921) versus streptokinase (preliminary data)

Mireille L. Brochier[1], B. Charbonnier[1], H. Kulbertus[2], P. Materne[2], B. Letac[3], A. Cribier[3], J. P. Monassier[4], A. Sacrez[5], and J. P. Favier[5]

[1] Department of Cardiology, CHU Trousseau, Tours (France),
[2] Institute of Medicine, Hôpital de Bavière, Liège (Belgium),
[3] Service de Cardiologie, CHU Rouen,
[4] Service de Cardiologie, CH Colmar, and
[5] Service de Cardiologie, CHU Strasbourg (France)

Acylated plasminogen streptokinase (SK) activator complex (APSAC or BRL 26921) differs from SK by 4 characteristics (6):
1. It is a direct activator complex of SK and lysyl-plasminogen.
2. Lysyl-plasminogen has a high affinity for fibrin.
3. The complex is temporarily inactivated by coupling an acyl group to its catalytic centre and following infusion, a plasminogen activator is generated by spontaneous deacylation of the complex.
4. The deacylation half life is 40 minutes and biological half life is particularly long (90 minutes) (5).

Therefore, it should have some advantages in acute myocardial infarction (AMI):
1. be easy to apply in an early intravenous bolus,
2. have a prolonged in situ fibrinolytic activity,
3. have a higher artery patency rate and a lower reocclusion rate than other fibrinolytic treatments.

The aims of our multicenter randomized study were:
1. to compare the early coronary angiography patency rate of either i.v. BRL 26921 or i.v. SK infusion in patients with AMI;
2. to monitor safety and tolerance for up to 24 hours after treatment.

Methods

Inclusion criteria were as normal:
1. patients 70 years of age or under,
2. patients admitted within 6 hours of a chest pain lasting more than 30 minutes, resistant to nitrates,
3. ECG ST segment elevation >1 mm in standard leads, >2 mm in chest leads,
4. no contraindications for angiography or thrombolysis.

Stratification between anterior and posterior AMI was performed before randomization and informed consent.

Patients then received either an intravenous bolus of 30 units of BRL 26921 or an intravenous infusion of 1.5 million units of SK for 1 hour.

Coronary angiogram was performed between the first and the fourth hour, about 90 minutes. The main endpoint was the patency rate of the infarct related artery. Only grades 2 and 3 of artery patency were considered as a success.

All patients received heparin after coronary angiogram when the fibrinogen level was equal to or above 1 g/liter.

Results

Seventy patients were involved in the study. Here we present the results of the first fifty patients (25 BRL and 25 SK). The patency rate was 76% in the BRL group, and 63% in the SK group.

Depending on the delay between treatment and angiography, there was a progression of patency rate from an early delay of less than 60 minutes, within the second hour and beyond the second hour, but the difference is not significant (Table 1). There was no difference in patency rate between anterior and inferior MI.

On the other hand, according to the delay between pain and treatment initiation, the shorter the delay the higher the patency rate (Table 2).

There was no significant difference between the fall in fibrinogen levels in the two groups (Fig. 1). Therefore, heparin could be administered from the eighteenth hour on average.

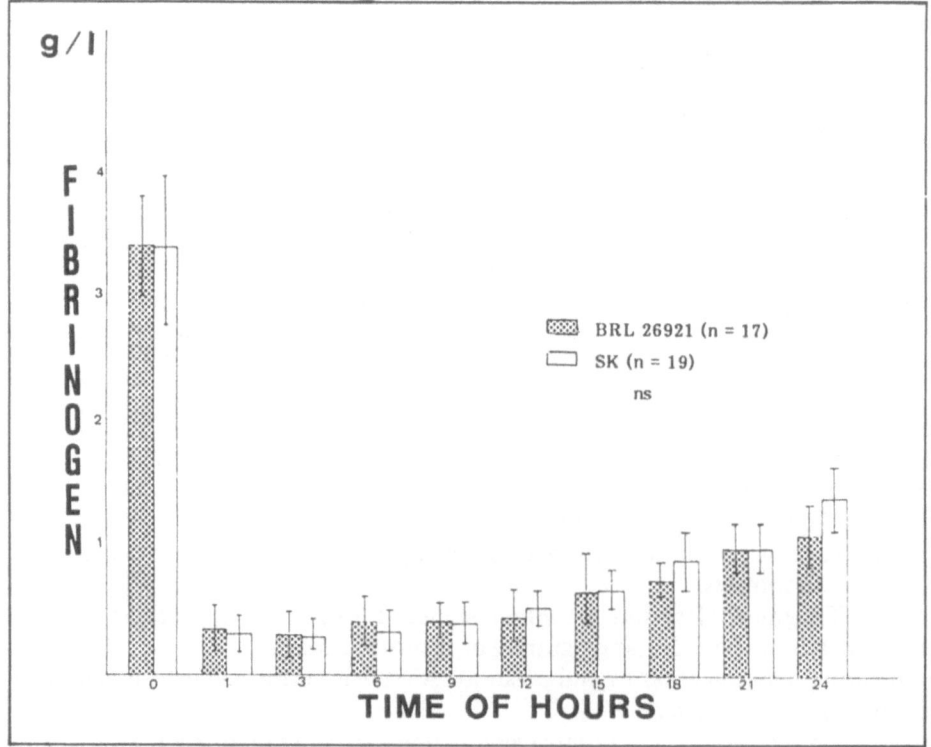

Fig. 1. Mean fibrinogen levels (±S.D.) in the two groups

Table 1. Patency assessment

Delay Trt./ angiography	BRL 26921		Streptokinase	
	Perfused (Gd. 2 & 3)	Not perfused (Gd. 0 & 1)	Perfused (Gd. 2 & 3)	Not perfused (Gd. 0 & 1)
≦ 60 min	4 (67%)	2	2 (33%)	4
60–120 min	12 (75%)	4	10 (71%)	4
> 120 min	3 (100%)	0	4 (80%)	1

Gd. = grade; Trt. = treatment

Table 2. Patency assessment

Delay pain/ treatment	BRL 26921		Streptokinase	
	Perfused (Gd. 2 & 3)	Not perfused (Gd. 0 & 1)	Perfused (Gd. 2 & 3)	Not perfused (Gd. 0 & 1)
≦ 3 h	10 (91%)	1	10 (66%)	5
3–6 h	9 (64%)	5	6 (60%)	4

Gd. = grade

The side effects were not severe during the first 24 hours, apart from a case of cerebrovascular accident in the BRL group, concerning a patient with a meningeal bleeding one year previously which had required surgery and one case of prolonged secondary hypotension which required dopamine (Table 3). Two patients died, one from cardiogenic shock on the second day and the other from a catheterization accident during a second coronary angiogram on the second day.

Two patients in each group required blood transfusion.

In a subgroup of this multicenter trial, 20 patients had three control angiograms at 90 minutes, 24 hours and in the 3rd week (Fig. 2). Patients of the BRL group had a 70%

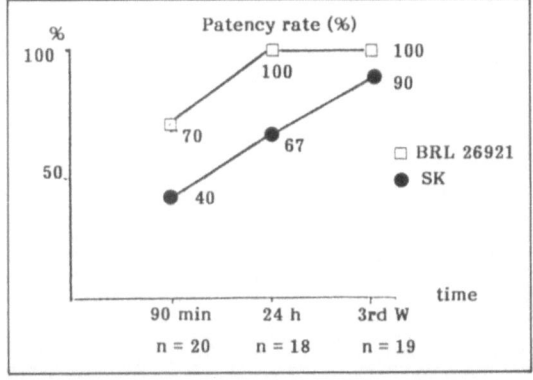

Fig. 2. Intravenous thrombolysis (BRL 26921 vs. SK) in acute myocardial infarction (subgroup of 20 pts with 3 angiography controls)

69

Table 3. Adverse events

Time	BRL 26921		SK	
	≦24 h	>24 h	≦24 h	>24 h
Haematoma	–	3 (1*)	1	2*
GI bleeding	–	1*	1	–
CVA	1	–	–	–
Hypotension	2	–	–	–
Other	4	–	–	–

* Transfusion required.
GI = gastrointestinal,   CVA = cerebrovascular   accident,   SK = streptokinase

patency rate at 90 minutes and a 100% patency rate at 24 h and in the 3rd week while patients of the SK group had patency rates of 40%, 67% and 90% respectively. Two patients out of 10 in the SK group had a controlled reocclusion, one within the first day, but the artery was patent in the 3rd week, and the other was patent in the 3rd week. In 12 patients without secondary percutaneous transluminal coronary angioplasty (PTCA), the residual stenosis was $70 \pm 29\%$ at 90 minutes, $64 \pm 28\%$ at 24 hours and $56 \pm 29\%$ in the third week ($p < .001$). In 5 patients with secondary PTCA, the residual stenosis was $77 \pm 15\%$, $47 \pm 15\%$ and $37 \pm 3\%$ respectively (NS). In this subgroup, the ejection fraction and the segmental ventricular kinetics were compared in 14 patients of the 2 groups at 24 hours and in the 3rd week. There was a difference between ejection fraction in the group of occluded arteries (0.48 vs. 0.58 $p < 0.05$ in the 3rd week) and a decrease in hypokinetic segment percentage between 24 h and the 3rd week (32% vs. 21% in patent arteries group –NS) (Fig. 3).

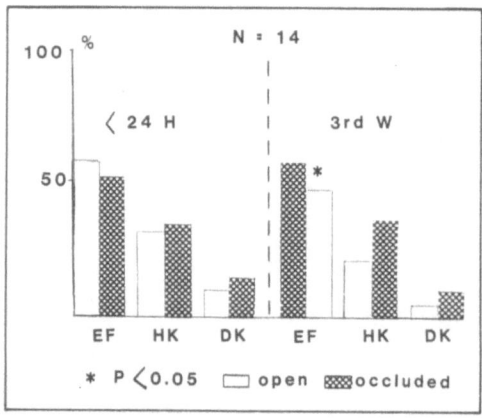

Fig. 3. Intravenous-thrombolysis (BRL 26921 vs. SK) in acute myocardial infarction: ejection fraction and wall motion (%)

Comments

Preliminary open and some controlled studies in the literature (1, 3, 7) had previously pointed out the high patency rate obtained with BRL 26921, including 2 studies with pre and post infusion coronary angiograms. And recently De Bono reported 75 cases of AMI treated with the same dose regimen and a patency rate of 89% at the 90 min coronary angiograms (2).

Finally APSAC has the advantage of a prolonged fibrinolytic activity (4) due to both long half life of 90 minutes and progressive deacylation. Therefore, it may be administered in a rapid early intravenous injection.

Conclusion

In the race against time of thrombolysis in acute myocardial infarction, one fact is that BRL 26921 has been found to give rapid reperfusion in the majority of cases treated with a single intravenous bolus injection without major side effect. Three other prospects need further investigations. They concern the likely thrombus specificity, the high percentage of early reperfusion, and the low risk of reocclusion due to the long biological half life.

References

1. Been M, de Bono DP, Hillis WS, Hornung R (1984) Coronary thrombolysis with i.v. BRL 26921, an acylated plasminogen streptokinase complex. Circulation 70 (Suppl II): abstract 1320
2. de Bono DP, Been M, Boulton F (1985) Acyenzyme BRL 26921 et thrombolyse coronarienne. Colloque de la Société Française d'Hématologie, Paris 26 October
3. de Wilde PH, Taeymans Y, de Moor D, Huyghens L, Block P (1985) L'emploi du BRL 26921 i.v. dans l'infarctus aigu du myocarde. 13th Congrès de Cardiologie de Langue Française. Fort de France, 9–11 December
4. Hoffmann JJML, Van Rey FJW, Bonnier JJRM (1985) Systemic effects of BRL 26921 during thrombolytic treatment of acute myocardial infarction. Thromb Res 37:567–572
5. Matsuo O, Collen D, Verstraete M (1981) On the fibrinolytic and thrombolytic properties of active site p anisoylated streptokinase-plasminogen complex (BRL 26921). Thromb Res 24:347–358
6. Smith RAG, Dupe RJ, English PD, Green J (1981) Fibrinolysis with acyl-enzymes: a new approach to thrombolytic therapy. Nature 290:505–508
7. Van Rey FJ, Bonnier HJ, Michels HR, Mamdouh IE, Hoffmann HJ (1984) Efficacy and safety of BRL 26921 a new fibrinolytic agent for i.v. administration in acute myocardial infarction. Circulation 70 (Suppl II): abstract 1319

Authors' address:
Professor Mireille Brochier
Department of Cardiology
CHU Trousseau
37044 Tours Cedex, France

Short and long term results with intracoronary SK with regard to further treatment and age of patients – experiences in Aachen –*

R. v. Essen, R. Uebis, W. Schmidt, R. Dörr, W. Merx, J. Meyer, S. Effert, P. Schweizer, R. Erbel, P. Bardos, C. Minale, and B. J. Messmer

Abteilung Innere Medizin I und Abteilung Herz- und Gefäßchirurgie der Rheinisch-Westfälischen Technischen Hochschule Aachen (West Germany)

Introduction

Twenty-five years ago Boucek and co-workers (4) described treatment with thrombolysin of eight patients who had suffered acute myocardial infarction. Using a catheter they introduced the drug directly into the sinus of Valsalva and could observe a return to normal within 6 h in the electrocardiograms of two patients. This was then followed in more extensive investigations (29) by systemic application of streptokinase in acute myocardial infarction. The results of eight randomised studies were published between 1969 and 1979 (1–3, 5, 7, 12–14). A significant drop in mortality could only be demonstrated in three of these studies with intravenous injection of streptokinase (5, 12, 13) and for this reason systemic streptokinase treatment was discontinued in most cardiology centres.

The "Renaissance" of streptokinase therapy in myocardial infarction began in 1978 with the intracoronary route of application (25–27). The then still controversial question of whether thrombus is the cause or the result of acute infarction has since been answered (35): in agreement with other groups we also found in 365 out of 461 patients (79%), who since March 1980 had undergone coronary angiography during the acute stage of infarction, thrombotic obstruction of the infarct vessel and a high degree of coronary stenosis in the remaining 96 (21%). We report our observations below.

Patients and methods

Between March 1980 and July 1984 (up until the start of the rt-plasminogen activator study) coronary angiography was performed immediately upon admission in all patients, regardless of age (387 men and 74 women), fitting the criteria listed in Table 1 who consented to the therapy and in whom there was no contraindication of streptokinase treatment. Premedication and dosage and duration of streptokinase therapy are given in Table 1.

Where the infarct vessel was partially obstructed streptokinase was infused for 30 min, but in the case of thrombotic obstruction and unsuccessful thrombolysis the treatment was stopped after 60 min. If the infarct vessel could be reopened success-

---

* Parts of these data have been published recently in the Deutsche Medizinische Wochenschrift by v. Essen et al. (9 b)

73

Table 1. Criteria for including patients in the study, streptokinase dosage, duration of lysis and premedication in selective thrombolysis

---

Acute myocardial infarction: ST elevation ≥ 0.3 mV in the case of anterior wall infarction and ≥ 0.2 mV in posterior wall infarction recorded within 8 h after onset

Streptokinase dosage: 3000 U/min until reperfusion, continued with 2000 U/min for at least 30 min. Duration of lysis in unsuccessful cases: 60 min

Other medication: 2–6 mg/h nitroglycerine, 200 mg Prednisolon, 10,000 U heparin, 1 g acetylsalicylic acid

---

fully the therapy was continued for a further 30 min. Subsequently angiography of the unaffected coronary arteries was performed. When reperfusion was achieved within 4 h after the onset of symptoms and multiple-vessel disease was revealed, bypass operation was then carried out (within the first ten days) and in the case of single-vessel disease, percutaneous transluminal coronary angioplasty (PTCA) was performed where possible in the same session (Fig. 1). At the end of the examination left ventricular angiography was performed in 30° RAO projection. All patients were subsequently heparinised (25,000–35,000 U/24 h i.v.) and treated further with nitroglycerine given parenterally (2–6 mg/h). The arterial introducer, which was left in position, allowed control angiography of the infarct vessel and left ventricular angiography to be performed on the third day. Patients who agreed to an invasive control investigation underwent angiography again 4–6 months later. After one year patients were examined in the Out Patients Department and over the following years records were kept of the subsequent course of all patients with the aid of questionnaires.

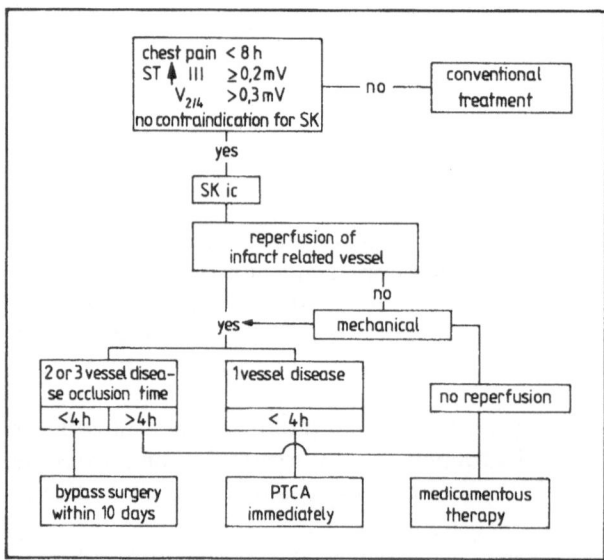

Fig. 1. Treatment of patients with acute myocardial infarction in relation to time of reperfusion

Table 2. Correlation between infarct vessel and success of thrombolysis

Infarct vessel	Patients n	Subtotal stenosis	Vessel occlusion	Unsuccess- ful lysis	Success- ful lysis
R. interventricularis anterior	212	49 (23%)	163 (77%)	21 (13%)	142 (87%)
Right coronary artery	175	34 (19%)	141 (81%)	10 (7%)	131 (93%)
R. circumflexus	61	12 (20%)	49 (80%)	14 (29%)	35 (71%)

Results

Coronary angiographic status before and after lysis therapy

Initial coronary angiography revealed a high degree of stenosis in 96 (21%) patients but no total occlusion of the vessels affected by the infarction (group A). In 365 patients (79%) there was complete occlusion of the infarct vessel. This could be reopened in 315 patients (86%; group B) but attempts at reperfusion were unsuccessful in 50 patients (14%; group C). Thus prior to thrombolysis, 79% of the infarct vessels were occluded and after thrombolysis only 11%.

Table 2 reflects the success of thrombolysis in relation to vessel localisation. The period of ischemia, i.e. the time from the onset of acute symptoms up until reperfusion of the infarct vessel as documented by coronary angiography was 213 ± 87 min. In the mean infarct vessels were reopened 24 min after the start of intracoronary streptokinase infusion.

Follow-up treatment after successful thrombolysis therapy

Early bypass operation was performed in the first 10 days in patients with multiple-vessel disease who had undergone successful recanalisation of the infarct vessel within 4 hours or in patients with initially open infarct vessel (n = 78). 163 patients had single-vessel disease and thus percutaneous transluminal coronary angioplasty (PTCA) was indicated in these patients. PTCA was successful in 129 of these 163 pa-

Table 3. Follow-up treatment of individual groups with PTCA, bypass operation or conservative therapy

	PTCA	Bypass	Conservative	Total
Group A Vessel initially open	25	18	53	96
Group B Successful lysis	104	60	151	315
Group C Unsuccessful lysis	0	0	50	50
Total	129	78	254	461

tients (79%; 104 patients from group B, 25 patients from group A), where success was taken to be an increase in diameter of more than 20%. In 96% of these patients vasodilatation was carried out directly following streptokinase infusion.

Conservative follow-up treatment without bypass operation and PTCA was given in altogether 254 patients. 50 of these patients belonged to group C, i.e. reperfusion of the infarct vessel was initially impossible. 53 patients had a primarily open infarct vessel. In 151 patients thrombolysis therapy was successful but PTCA was impossible or unsuccessful, or a bypass operation had not been carried out in the early stage in patients with multiple-vessel disease because of an occlusion time of more than 4 hours (Table 3).

Mortality after successful thrombolysis

a) Early mortality: The 30-day mortality rate was 7.8% (n = 16) in the 204 patients from groups A and B who had undergone conservative follow up therapy and 7 (14%) of the 50 patients with unsuccessful thrombolysis (group C) died. Four of the 129 patients with successful PTCA died (3.1%).

The lowest mortality rate was seen in the 78 patients with short occlusion time and early bypass operation, only two of whom died on the 2nd day after the operation. The mean age of the patients did not vary significantly in the individual subgroups (Table 4).

The cause of death in altogether 29 patients was heart failure or cardiogenic shock in 20 cases, tachycardiac dysrhythmia unresponsive to therapy in 3 cases, pulmonary embolism in one case and postoperative haemorrhage in another case. Two patients died of unexplained causes.

Rupture of the heart occurred in only three patients. Two of these patients died – in one the infarct vessel could not be reperfused. The third patient suffered rupture of the free wall of the left ventricle a few minutes after the start of streptokinase infusion but by immediate pericardial tap the cardiac tamponade could be cleared and the patient saved.

b) Long-term prognosis: Table 4 shows the mortality rate after 1 year in the different groups, revealing the highest level in the group receiving conservative treatment at 21.2%. We were able to follow up 163 of the conservatively treated patients for up

Table 4. Mortality rates after 30 days and 1 year depending on follow-up treatment after successful and unsuccessful thrombolysis

	Age (years)		Mortality rate after	
	$x \pm s$	range	30 days	1 year
Conservative follow-up treatment (n = 204)	57 ± 12	21–83	7.8%	21.2%
PTCA (n = 129)	56 ± 10	34–76	3.1%	9.3%
Bypass operation (early) (n = 78)	56 ± 7	39–76	2.6%	6.4%
Unsuccessful lysis (n = 50)	54 ± 9	34–79	14.0%	20.0%

to 22 months after the treatment. The 43 patients with an initially open vessel had a significantly better prognosis (11%) than the 120 patients with an initially closed vessel (18%; P < 0.05, "Fischer's exact test").

Subgroup of elderly patients

Altogether 56 of the patients were 70 years and older (70–84, mean 73.4, 44 men and 11 women). Thrombolysis treatment was without success in 15 patients from this group, while reperfusion of the infarct vessel was obtained in 41. 27 of these patients then received conservative follow up treatment, 11 PTCA treatment and in 3 a bypass operation was carried out (Fig. 2). The cause of death during the first year in

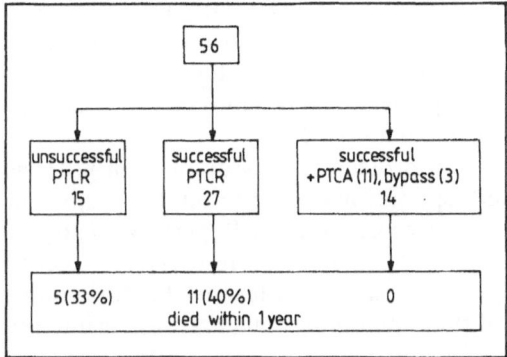

Fig. 2. Long-term prognosis in elderly patients depending on the success of thrombolysis or the subsequent bypass operation or PTCA (PTCR = percutaneous transluminal coronary reperfusion)

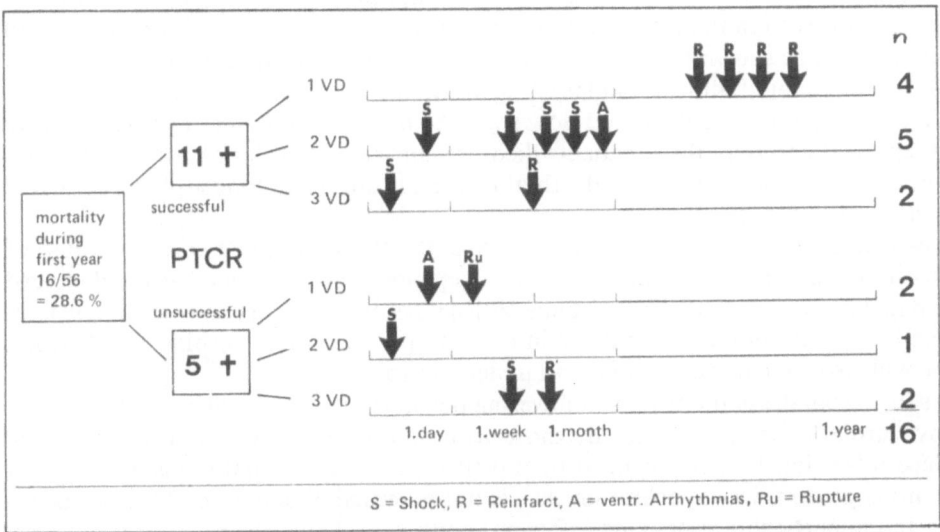

Fig. 3. Cause and time of deaths in patients aged 70 years and over in regard to successful or unsuccessful PTCR (PTCR = percutaneous transluminal coronary reperfusion; VD = vessel disease)

regard to successful or unsuccessful thrombolysis and the status of the coronary arteries (1 VD = one vessel disease, 2 VD = two vessel disease, 3 VD = three vessel disease) are listed in Fig. 3).

Discussion

The intracoronary application of streptokinase with visualization of thrombolysis directly in the infarct vessel made it possible to record the effect of reperfusion on clinical state, electrocardiograms and myocardial function. The clinical improvement of the patients is often dramatic especially with regard to pain. This correlates with the rapid disappearance of ST-segment elevation which is evidence of good restoration of blood flow to the infarct area (10). In some cases complete normalisation of the defective ventricular function was observed and patients suffering cardiogenic shock could be saved (11, 19, 24a). Both the results presented here and those of other authors (20, 30) are evidence that reperfusion is possible in a high percentage of patients using intracoronary application of streptokinase and that it can even be further improved by additional mechanical manipulation (32, 33).

The two basic questions whether reperfusion protects myocardium from necrosis and whether streptokinase application and reperfusion are dangerous for the patient can be answered, based on our six years' experience, as follows: Reperfusion can preserve ischaemic myocardium from necrosis. The extent of preservation depends among other things upon the localization of the site of occlusion, the duration of ischaemia, whether there is residual blood flow and on the collateral vessels into the infarct region.

Apart from mainly localised, easily controllable bleeding and haematomas at the puncture site in 7.4% (21) of our patients there were no complications arising from streptokinase. Rupture of the heart, a fatal complication following acute infarction, is, in contrast to initial fears, rare rather than common following thrombolysis and reperfusion, as shown by the results (9a). Atrioventricular blocks disappear on reperfusion. A rapid idioventricular compensation rhythm occurs temporarily in 20–30% of the patients as the blood flow begins to be restored. Later, dysrhythmias are exceptional and only three patients died of ventricular fibrillation a few days after successful thrombolysis. Thus, dysrhythmias and rupture no longer play a large role as a cause of death.

Death in consequence of pumping failure is the third and most common cause of death in acute infarction and is crucially dependent on the extent of the damaged and no longer contractile myocardium. When it becomes possible to save enough ischaemic myocardium by reperfusion in order to prevent severe cardiac insufficiency, we will also have this cause of death under control.

As seen from the point of view of lowering the mortality rate, patients with extensive myocardial infarction, especially those with anterior wall infarction or second or third infarction, benefit the most by this therapy, provided that ischaemic myocardium is present, i.e. myocardium that is not irreversibly damaged. This can be expected in particular in patients suffering severe pain. From the point of view of detecting an improvement in cardiac function, in particular of the reduction of the ischaemic area of the left ventricle involved in contraction, the duration of ischaemia (occlusion time) is of course of crucial importance. Although already after an occlusion time of 2 h in some cases no improvement of the regional wall movement impairment by reperfusion can be demonstrated, there are patients who even after an occlusion time of 5–6 h show recovery of areas of myocardium. Anterior and posterior wall infarction have different characteristics. Depending on vascularisation the anterior wall generally has a shorter tolerance of ischaemia than the posterior wall (28). In a relatively large number of patients we were unable to show echocardiographically any significant improvement in ventricular function where ischaemia duration was more than 4 h (18, 31). Mathey and co-workers (21) also found a substantial improvement of regional wall movement impairment only in conjunction with a short ischaemia time using left ventricular cine-angiography.

To assume from this, however, that an attempt at reperfusion is no longer worthwhile after 3–4 h is, after what has been said above, open to problems and can at best be understood from the point of view of obtaining an "objective" demonstration of an improvement in contraction. (The limited information provided by echocardiograms and ventriculograms in quantifying the impaired heart muscle must be taken into account here.) In patients with severe symptoms (pain and dyspnoea), especially in those with anterior wall infarction, we would begin reperfusion even after 4 h in order to improve the prognosis. The question, up to what age patients with acute infarction should be given thrombolysis, is closely related to the question of what therapy should be given as a follow up to thrombolysis therapy.

The long-term protection of myocardium saved by early thrombolysis was the main aspect which in 1980 led us to introduce in our clinic dilatation (24) in the case of single-vessel disease and operation (23) in the case of multiple-vessel disease with ischaemia time under 4 h. As with advancing age the probability of multiple-vessel disease seems to increase and as a bypass operation can only really be considered for biologically younger patients over 70, thrombolysis in this age group already becomes difficult from this point of view. As Fig. 2 demonstrates the mortality rate after one year for elderly patients who have received thrombolysis alone is even higher at 37% than that of patients in whom recanalization of the infarct vessel was unsuccessful (29%). While the still relatively low figures only allow provisional conclusions to be made, thrombolysis therapy alone without subsequent long-term securing of reperfusion by PTCA or bypass operation (none of the 14 patients treated in this way died) seems to have little point with regard to mortality in this age group in particular. Also in the group as a whole better results were obtained in patients who subsequently underwent coronary vasodilatation or bypass operation (Table 4). At 8% the mortality rate within the first 30 days in all patients in whom treatment was initially successful was about as low as that obtained by Kennedy (15). When patients over 70 are excluded the mortality was even as low as 5% in our group.

The data show that in the case of acute myocardial infarction, prognosis can be fundamentally improved if, according to the state of the coronary vessels in individual patients, thrombolysis is followed up by optimal revascularisation. Indication for further treatment should be based on among other things the patients' symptoms and the objective evidence of ischaemia. It is still doubtful whether the long-term prognosis is significantly better following thrombolysis treatment alone than after conventional therapy. If placebo controlled studies using intravenous streptokinase with no further measures for reperfusion, as are presently being repeated, do not lead to a significant drop in mortality, one cannot infer from this that thrombolysis therapy is ineffective in acute myocardial infarction (particularly as intravenous application of streptokinase apparently only induces rapid thrombolysis in 50% of patients). The therapy for acute infarction is, however, limited by the high technical and personnel costs (8). It is thus our aim in the next phase of this study to establish what patients would profit most from these revascularisation measures.

At present new thrombolytic substances are undergoing first clinical trials (rt-plasminogen activator (rt-PA), acyl-streptokinase plasminogen, pro-urokinase) (6, 16, 17, 34). These drugs are expected to produce as high a rate of reperfusion as intracoronary application of streptokinase, but they have the great advantage that they can be given intravenously and unlike streptokinase in high doses do not lead to activation of the whole coagulation system with the usual complications of haemorrhaging. The multi-centre European co-operation in studies with rt-PA has now been completed and a similar investigation has been carried out in the United States (TIMI study). It is conceivable that these substances will in future be in use in general hospitals, and that after successful reperfusion patients would then be sent to specialised centres for further treatment (PTCA or bypass) to ensure long-term coronary blood flow.

It can no longer be doubted that reopening of the infarct vessel has brought about a turning point in infarct treatment. In the next few years it will be our aim to make this therapy as effective and safe as possible and thus to make it generally practicable. After the vessel has been successfully reopened, early securing of the initial success by measures guaranteeing long-term coronary blood flow is the logical consequence, as also shown by experience with chronic coronary heart disease.

Acknowledgements

The results presented here would not have been possible without the devoted effort of the doctors and nurses of the intensive care unit, the technicians and nurses of the cardiac catheterization unit and the outstanding co-operation of the surrounding hospitals. We would like to take this opportunity to thank them all.

References

1. Aber CP, Bas NM, Berry CL, Carson PHM, Dobbs RJ, Fox KM, Hamblin JJ, Haydu SP, Howitt G, MacIver JE, Portal RW, Raftery EB, Rousell RH, Stock JPP (1976) Streptokinase in acute myocardial infarction. A controlled multicentre study in the United Kingdom. Br Med J 2:1100
2. Amery A, Roeber G, Vermeulen HJ, Verstraete M (1969) Single-blind randomized multicentre trial comparing heparin and streptokinase treatment in recent myocardial infarction. Acta Med Scand 505 (Suppl):5
3. Bett JHN, Castaldi PA, Chesterman CN, Hale GS, Hirsh J, Isbister JP, McDonald IG, McLean KH, Morgan JJ, O'Sullivan EF, Rosenbaum M (1973) Australian multicentre trial of streptokinase in acute myocardial infarction. Lancet I:57
4. Boucek RJ, Murphy WP Jr, Sommer LS, Voudoukis IJ (1960) Segmental perfusion of the coronary arteries with fibrinolysin in man following a myocardial infarction. Am J Cardiol 6:525

5. Breddin K, Ehrly AM, Fechler L, Frick D, König H, Kraft H, Krause H, Krywanek HJ, Kut-schera J, Lösch HW, Ludwig O, Mikat B, Rausch F, Rosenthal P, Sartory S, Voigt G (1973) Die Kurzzeitfibrinolyse beim akuten Myokardinfarkt. Dtsch Med Wschr 98:861
6. Collen D, Topol EJ, Tiefenbrunn AJ, Gold HK, Weisfeldt ML, Sobel BE, Leinbach RC, Brinker JA, Ludbrook PA, Yasuda I, Bulkley BH, Robinson AK, Hutter AM Jr, Bell WR, Spadaro JJ Jr, Khaw BA, Grossbard EB (1984) Coronary thrombolysis with recombinant human tissue-type plasminogen activator. A prospective, randomized, placebo-controlled trial. Circulation 70:1012
7. Dioguardi N, Mannucci PM, Lotto A, Rossi P, Levi GF, Lomanto B, Rota M, Mattei G, Proto C, Fiorelli G (1971) Controlled trial of streptokinase and heparin in acute myocardial infarction. Lancet II:891
8. Dörr R, Essen R v, Ahnert F, Tolxdorff T (1984) Financial background of transluminal coronary recanalization MCR and regional distribution of cardiac catheterization laboratories in the Federal Republic of Germany. Eur Heart J, 5. Suppl 1:24 (Abstr)
9a. Essen R v, Effert S (1980) Herzruptur. Dtsch Med Wschr 105:495
9b. Essen R v, Uebis R, Schmidt W, Dörr R, Merx W, Meyer J, Effert F, Schweizer P, Erbel R, Bardos T, Minale C, Messmer BJ (1985) Intrakoronare Streptokinase beim akuten Herzinfarkt. Dtsch Med Wschr 110:570–575
10. Essen R v, Merx W, Schweizer P, Bethge Ch, Effert S (1982) Elektrokardiographische Zeichen einer erfolgreichen Thrombolyse durch intrakoronare Streptokinaseinfusion beim akuten Myokardinfarkt. Z Kardiol 71:147
11. Essen R v, Lambertz H, Schmidt W, Rustige I, Uebis R, Effert S (1984) Successful recanalization of a left main coronary artery occlusion. Amer J Cardiol 53:356
12. European Cooperative Study Group for Streptokinase Treatment in Acute Myocardial Infarction (1979) Streptokinase in acute myocardial infarction. New Engl J Med 301:797
13. European Working Party (1971) Streptokinase in recent myocardial infarction. A controlled multicentre trial. Br Med J 3:325
14. Heikinheimo R, Ahrenberg P, Honkapohja H, Lisalo E, Kallio V, Konttinen Y, Leskinen O, Mustahiemi H, Reinikainen M, Siitonen L (1971) Fibrinolytic treatment in acute myocardial infarction. Acta Med Scand 189:7
15. Kennedy JW, Ritchie JL, Davies KB, Fritz JK (1983) Western Washington randomized trial of intracoronary streptokinase in acute myocardial infarction. New Engl J Med 309:1477
16. Laffel GL, Braunwald E (1984) Thrombolytic therapy. A new strategy for the treatment of acute myocardial infarction (Part one). New Engl J Med 311:710
17. Laffel GL, Braunwald E (1984) Thrombolytic therapy. A new strategy for the treatment of acute myocardial infarction (Part two). New Engl J Med 311:776
18. Lambertz H, Schweizer P, Krebs W, Merx W, Erbel R, Essen R v, Uebis R, Erckelens F v, Meyer J, Effert S (1984) Echokardiographische Verlaufskontrolle des akuten Myokardinfarktes nach intrakoronarer Streptolysebehandlung. Z Kardiol 73:321
19. Mathey DG, Kuck KH, Remmecke J, Tilsner V, Bleifeld W (1980) Transluminal recanalization of coronary artery thrombosis. A preliminary report of its application in cardiogenic shock. Eur Heart J 1:207
20. Mathey DG, Schofer J, Bleifeld W (1984) Intrakoronare Thrombolyse – eine bereits gesicherte Therapie des akuten Herzinfarktes? Dtsch Med Wschr 109:678
21. Mathey DG, Sheehan FH, Schofer J, Bleifeld W, Dodge HT (1982) Left ventricular function following intracoronary thrombolysis in acute myocardial infarction. Circulation 66 (Suppl II):335
22. Merx W, Dörr R, Rentrop P, Blanke H, Karsch KR, Mathey DG, Kremer P, Rutsch W, Schmutzler H (1981) Evaluation of the effectiveness of intracoronary streptokinase infusion in acute myocardial infarction. Postprocedure management and hospital course in 204 patients. Am Heart J 102:1181
23. Messmer BJ, Merx W, Meyer J, Bardos P, Minale C, Effert S (1983) New developments in medical-surgical treatment of acute myocardial infarction. Ann Thorac Surg 35:70
24. Meyer J, Merx W, Schmitz H, Erbel R, Kiesslich T, Dörr R, Lambertz H, Bethge C, Krebs W, Bardos P, Minale C, Messmer BJ, Effert S (1982) Percutaneous transluminal coronary

angioplasty immediately after intracoronary streptolysis of transmural myocardial infarction. Circulation 66:905

24a. M J, Merx W, Dörr R, Lambertz H, Bethge C, Effert S (1982) Successful treatment of acute myocardial infarction shock by combined percutaneous transluminal coronary recanalization (PTCR) and percutaneous transluminal coronary angioplasty (PTCA). Am Heart J 103:132

25. Neuhaus KL, Bornikoel K, Tebbe U, Kreuzer H (1979) Beseitigung eines akuten thrombotischen Koronarverschlusses durch Kathetermanöver. Z Kardiol 68:298

26. Rentrop P, de Vivie ER, Karsch KR, Kreuzer H (1978) Acute coronary occlusion with impending infarction as an angiographic complication relieved by guide-wire recanalization. Clin Cardiol 1:101

27. Rentrop P, Blanke H, Wiegand V, Karsch KR (1979) Wiedereröffnung verschlossener Kranzgefäße im akuten Infarkt mit Hilfe von Kathetern. Transluminale Rekanalisation. Dtsch Med Wschr 104:1401

28. Schmidt WG, Merx W, Essen R v, Uebis R, Effert S, Schmidt-Wenz R (1984) Determinants of infarct size in patients successfully treated by intracoronary thrombolysis. Texas Heart Inst J 11:260

29. Schmutzler R, Heckner F, Körtge P, van de Loo J, Pezold FA, Poliwoda H, Praetorius F, Zekorn D (1966) Zur thrombolytischen Therapie des frischen Herzinfarktes. 1. Einführung, Behandlungspläne, allgemeine klinische Ergebnisse. Dtsch Med Wschr 91:581

30. Schwarz F, Kübler W (1984) Thrombolytische Therapie des akuten Herzinfarktes. Internist (Berl.) 25:713

31. Schweizer P, Merx W, Erbel R, Erckelens H v, Krebs W, Lambertz H, Meyer J, Effert S (1982) Echokardiographische Kontrolle des akuten Myokardinfarktes vor und nach Streptolysebehandlung. Z Kardiol 71:155

32. Uebis R, Essen R v, Merx W, Schmidt WG, Emons HP, Effert S (1984) Combined medical and mechanical recanalization versus superselective streptokinase alone. Reperfusion rate and time of occlusion. Circulation 70 (Suppl II):329

33. Uebis R, Essen R v, Merx W, Emons HP, Schmidt WG, Bertram B, Effert S (1984) Facilities to improve reperfusion rate and to decrease occlusion time in acute myocardial infarction. Eur Heart J 5 (Suppl I):163 (Abstr)

34. Van de Werf F, Ludbrook PA, Bergman SR, Tiefenbrunn AJ, Fox KAA, deGeest H, Verstraete M, Collen D, Sobel BE (1984) Coronary thrombolysis with tissue-type plasminogen activator in patients with evolving myocardial infarction. New Engl J Med 310:609

35. DeWood MA, Spores J, Notske R, Mouser LT, Burroughs R, Golden MS, Lang HT (1980) Prevalence of total coronary occlusion during the early hours of transmural myocardial infarction. New Engl J Med 303:897

Authors' address:

PD Dr. med R. von Essen
Stiftsklinik Augustinum
Klinik für Innere Medizin, Medizinische Klinik B
Wolkerweg 16
8000 Munich 70
West Germany

ECG and ECG mapping in myocardial infarction: facilities and limitations for assessment of coronary reperfusion therapy

W. G. Schmidt, R. v. Essen, R. Uebis, J. Silny, B. Vondenbusch, S. Effert, and G. Rau

Department of Internal Medicine I, RWTH Aachen and Helmholtz Institut für Biomedizinische Technik, Aachen (West Germany)

The diagnostic facilities of electrocardiography have been improved in recent years by the application of computer systems. Compared to conventional ECG recording, advantages result from the increased number of electrodes possible (precordial mapping ECG) and facilities to record continuously during a long period of up to several days.

There are well-suited applications in the field of reperfusion therapy in acute myocardial infarction. The time course of ST segment elevation during reperfusion therapy can be studied as well as changes of the QRS complex (4, 8, 9).

Methods

Precordial mapping system with 48 electrodes

A map with 48 equidistantly distributed electrodes is used. The diameter of the electrodes is 7 mm, the distance between electrodes is 35 mm. Signals from all electrodes can be recorded simultaneously by a computer system or by a conventional ECG recorder with a selection switch. Recording is standardised so that the upper left electrode of the map always lies within the second right intercostal space (1–3).

Improved system with 63 electrodes

The improved version of the mapping equipment, which has been developed at the Helmholtz Institute for Biomedical Technology in Aachen has several advantages:
– The electrodes are not made of metal, but of carbon reinforced resin material which is radiolucent and thus can be used even during catheterization studies as in PTCA or intracoronary thrombolysis procedures (Fig. 1).
– The system uses 63 electrodes. The distribution of the electrodes is nonequidistant. It results from spatial Fourier transform calculations and allows interpolation of up to 117 signals from these electrodes (9) (Fig. 2).

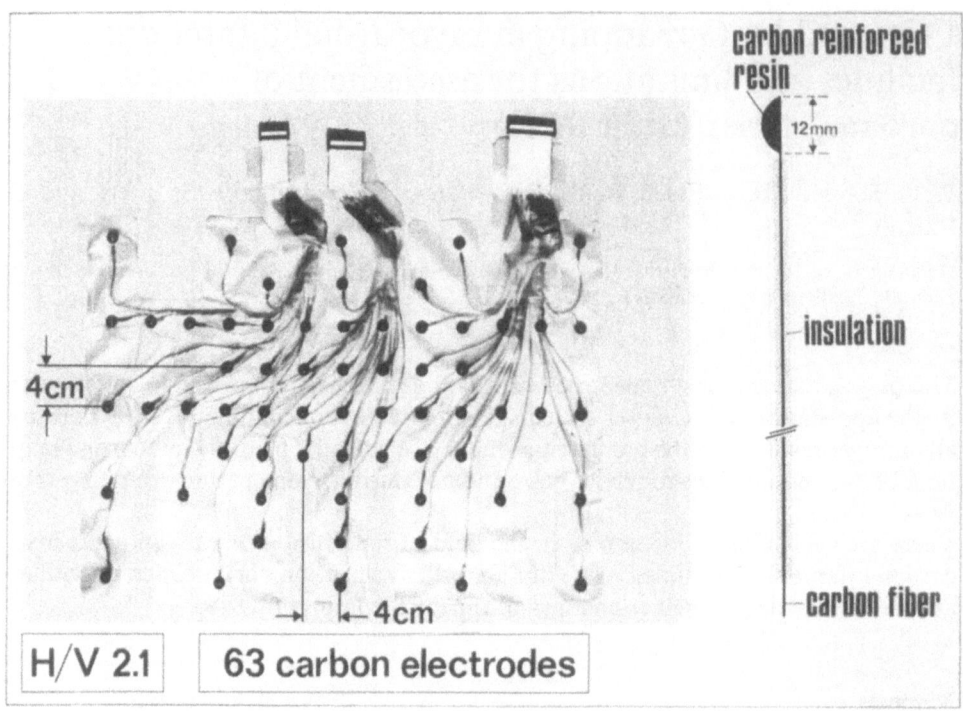

Fig. 1. Precordial mapping recording system with 63 non-equidistantly distributed electrodes. Electrodes are made from radiolucent resin material

Results

1. Application during thrombolysis

Figure 3 shows our findings in a patient with acute myocardial infarction in whom intracoronary thrombolysis and subsequent PTCA were performed. The first coronary angiography was performed 2 h and 15 min after the onset of chest pain. At this time pain was less severe than at the beginning of the attack. The LAO was severely narrowed but not completely occluded and ST segments were hardly elevated. During preparation for intracoronary infusion and PTCA, the patient reported an increase in chest pain and the LAD was now found completely occluded with a corresponding increase in ST segment elevation in the ECG. The vessel could be reopened by intracoronary infusion and subsequent PTCA. During ballon inflation the diagonal branches were temporarily occluded, too. This resulted in a further increase in ST segment elevation, not only in amplitude but also in spatial distribution and was now accompanied by a ST depression in the inferior leads. After the procedure the ST segments returned to normal and the residual stenosis of the vessel was abolished.

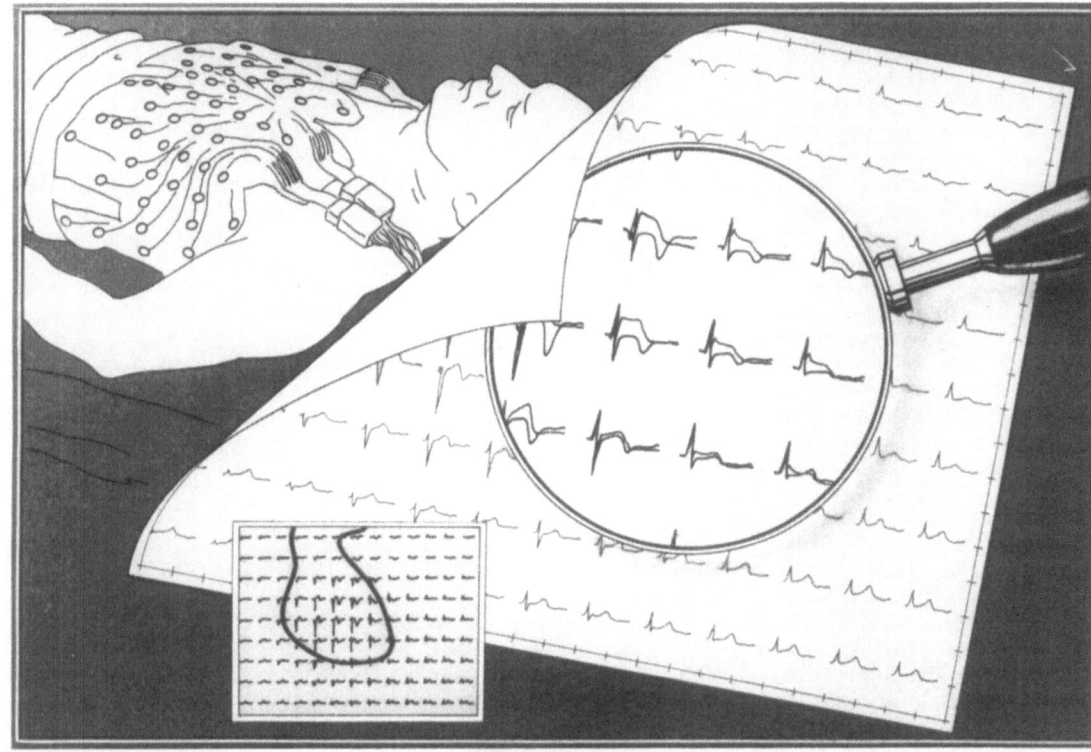

Fig. 2. Application of the recording map. *Left*: Position of the map applied to the patient. *Right*: Example of recording (two successive recordings are superimposed)

2. Development of ST segment elevation during reperfusion therapy

Recording of the ST segment elevation can also be obtained from the limb leads. Figure 4 shows the results of a group of patients either with anterior or inferior infarction. The sum of the absolute values of ST segment deviation from zero in all limb leads was calculated and showed a significant decrease after successful thrombolysis ($p < 0.05$) whereas it did not change if the vessel remained occluded or was already patent at the initial coronary angiography.

3. Long-term development of R wave amplitudes after thrombolysis

In this study 58 patients were examined who were treated by intracoronary thrombolysis for acute myocardial infarction (4,8). They were separated into four groups according to the results of therapy. The data could be compared with corresponding recordings from a group of 12 conventionally treated patients.

The totalled R wave amplitudes in all 48 leads of the initial recordings were compared with those after four months. Patients with severe narrowing of the infarct related vessel but without complete occlusion showed the best preserved R wave am-

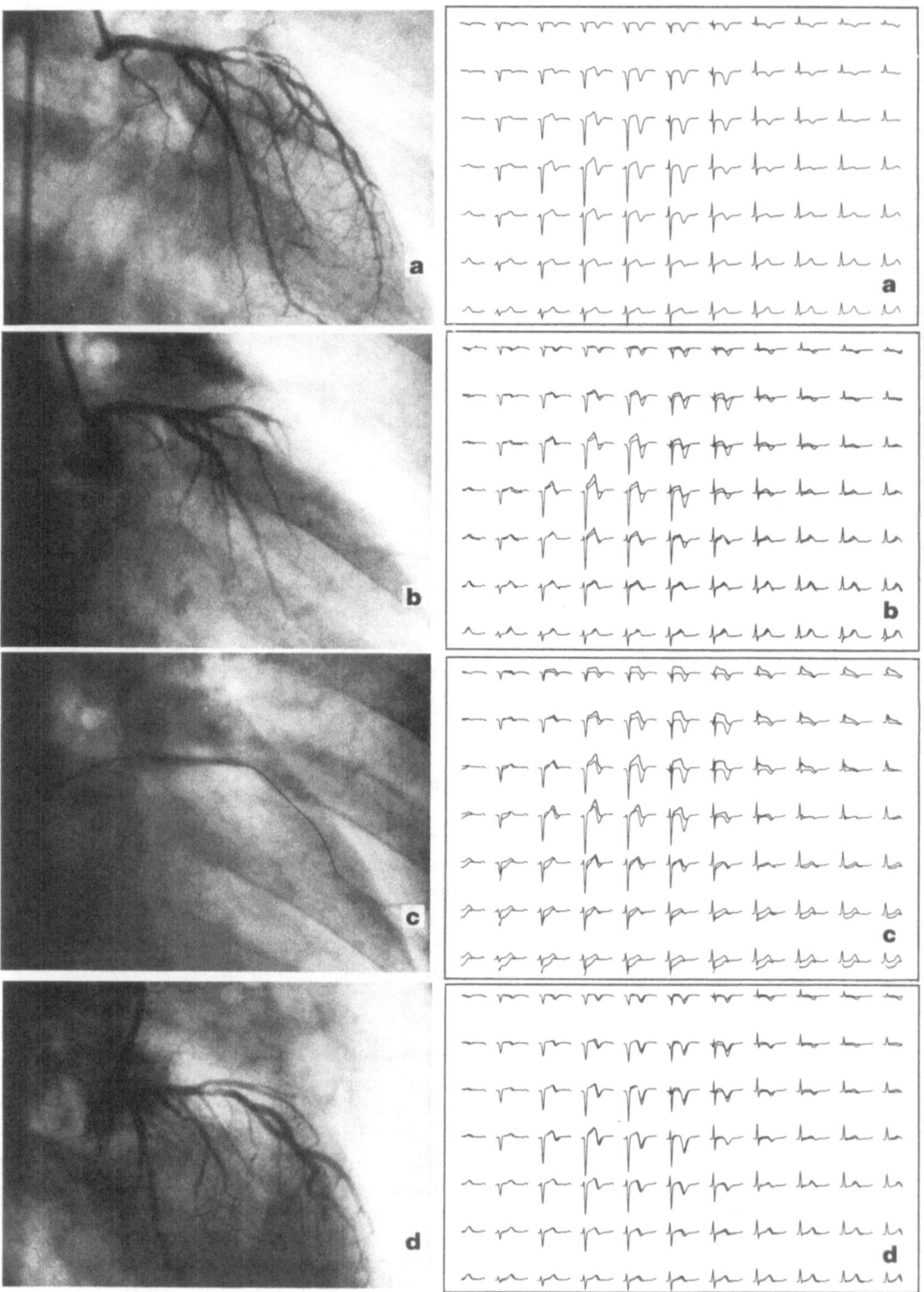

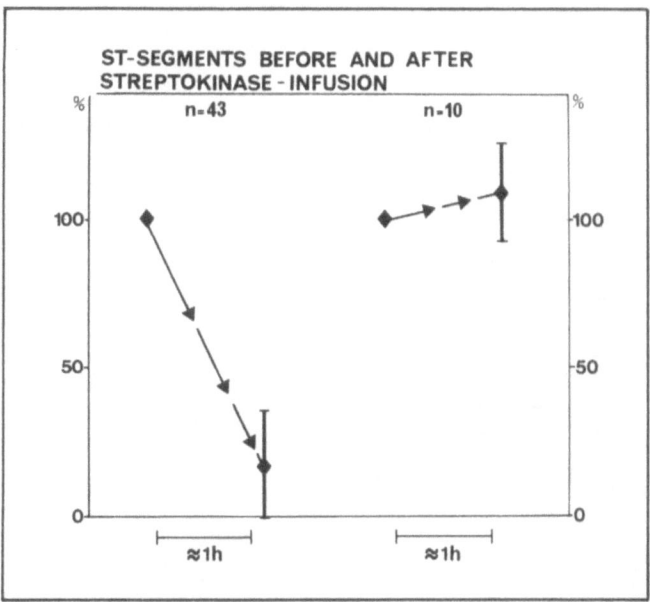

Fig. 4. Sum of ST segment deviation from zero in leads I, II, III in 53 patients with thrombolysis as percent of the initial value. A significant decrease can be seen in patients with successful reperfusion (*left*), no change occurs in patients with subtotal stenosis or occlusion without reperfusion (4)

plitudes of all groups and showed a further significant increase up to the fourth month thereafter. Patients with complete occlusion but successful reopening of the vessel showed a significant increase of R wave amplitudes as well. In the groups with conventional therapy or thrombolysis without success no significant changes occurred. Patients with reocclusion of a successfully treated vessel within the observation period showed a further significant decrease of R wave amplitude (Fig. 5).

The spatial distribution of these changes is shown in Fig. 6. It shows the average R wave changes in the group without thrombolysis treatment for all 48 electrode sides. In patients with subtotal occlusion increase of R waves can be seen at all sites, in cases with reocclusion, a further deterioration of the R wave amplitudes was found at all recording sites. This change was most pronounced in the upper left region. This would have been missed by recording with conventional Wilson lead systems.

Discussion

After reperfusion of an occluded coronary artery the initially elevated ST segments return to normal within a few minutes. Thus, reduction of the ST segment elevation

Fig. 3. Example of mapping ECG recording in acute anterior myocardial infarction. *Left*: Coronary angiography. *Right*: Mapping record (central section only), from b to d superimposed on the initial recording. *a* First angiography, LAD severely stenosed, but not occluded, *b* spontaneous occlusion of the vessel during streptokinase infusion, *c* PTCA balloon insufflation, *d* after successful reperfusion. For details see text

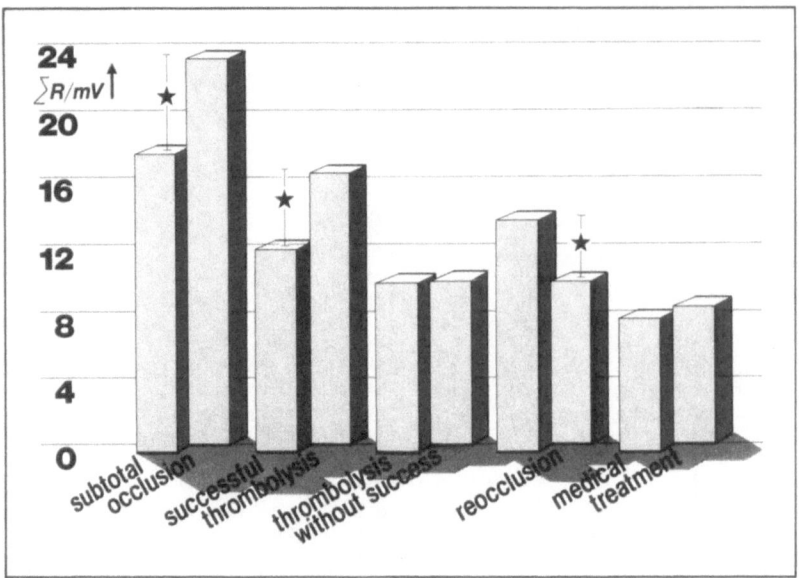

Fig. 5. Sum of R wave amplitudes in 48 precordial ECG recordings immediately after thrombolysis (*left columns*) as compared to 4 months thereafter (*right columns*). A significant ($p < 0.05$) increase is found in patients with subtotal stenosis or successful thrombolysis. Reocclusion of the vessel leads to a further significant loss of R waves

can be looked upon as a marker of reperfusion. Noninvasive markers of successful reperfusion will become more and more important with the widespread application of intravenous thrombolysis. Reperfusion can best be evaluated in continuous ECG recordings. Our recording system is well suited for this purpose. The possibility of reducing the number of electrodes without loss of information will have to be examined in order to make the system less expensive for widespread application.

The sum of R wave amplitudes and the number of Q waves can be used to evaluate ventricular function in patients with coronary artery disease. It can be obtained less expensively and more simply than any other parameter of ventricular function. For this, score systems have been developed to evaluate the ejection fraction of the left ventricle from standard ECG recordings (7, 10). Despite many different influencing factors, a significant correlation can be found. As expected, however, the prognostic predictive value of QRS score values is inferior as compared to ejection fraction (5, 6).

The diagnostic facilities of electrocardiography can be improved by application of precordial ECG mapping. This technique shows a better spatial resolution than conventional ECG and is well suited for intraindividual control studies, because of excellent reproducibility of the electrode positions, as our results show.

The further evolution of R wave amplitudes after myocardial infarction depends on the result of reperfusion therapy. An increase of R wave amplitudes after thrombo-

Fig. 6. Spatial distribution of R wave changes. The columns represent the difference in R wave amplitude between the acute stage of infarction and 4 months thereafter

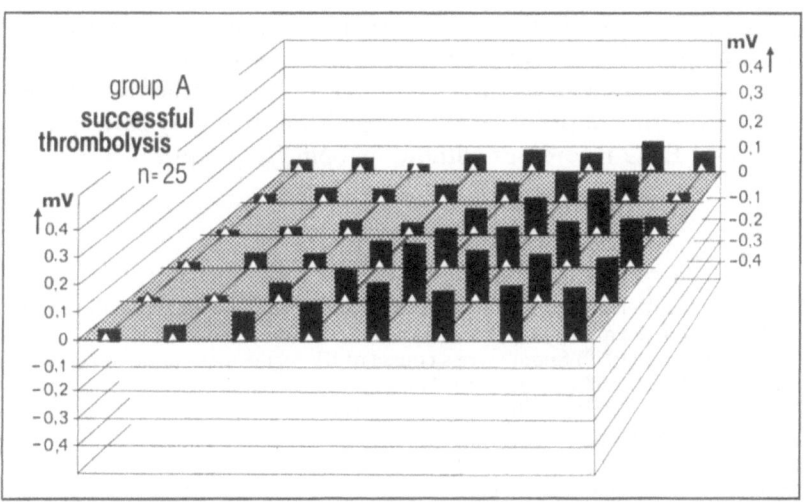

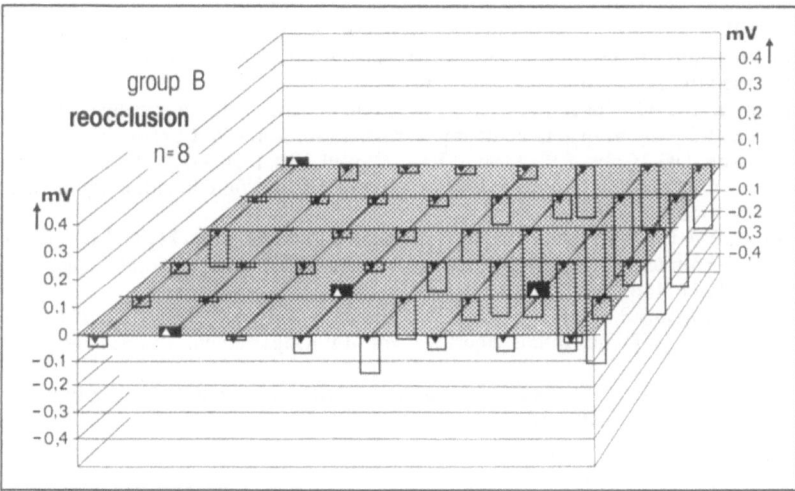

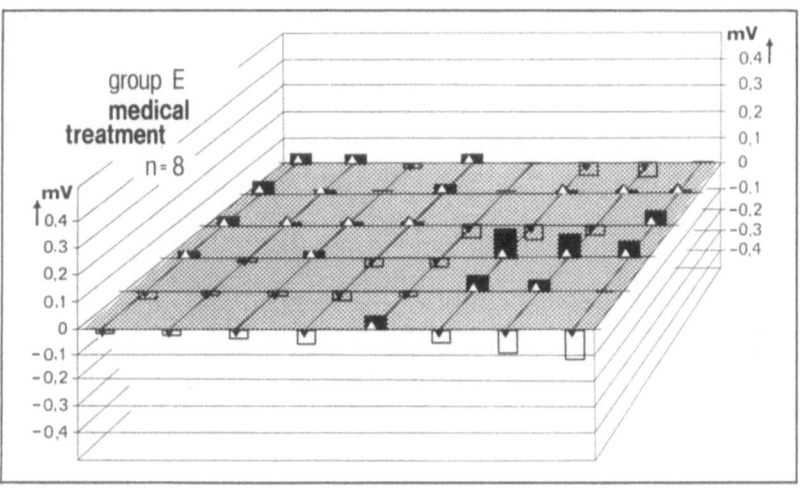

lysis can be expected if the vessel is successfully reperfused and remains open. So, reduction of R wave amplitude is not a definite sign of necrosis. Recovery may occur to some extent if reperfusion is achieved. Reocclusion leads to a further R wave decrease. The spatial distribution of the observed changes show that only part of them can be seen in standard ECG recordings without mapping techniques.

References

1. Essen R v, Merx W, Krebs W, Hanrath P, Silny J, Effert S (1977) Multiple Brustwandableitungen zur Verlaufsbeurteilung des akuten Myokardinfarktes. Z Kardiol 66:473–476
2. Essen R v, Merx W, Effert S (1979) Spontaneous course of ST-segment elevation in acute anterior myocardial infarction. Circulation 59:105–112
3. Essen R v, Merx W, Dörr R, Effert S, Silny J, Rau G (1980) QRS mapping in the evaluation of acute anterior myocardial infarction. Circulation 62:266–276
4. Essen R v, Schmidt W, Uebis R, Edelmann B, Effert S, Silny J, Rau G (1985) Myocardial infarction and thrombolysis. Electrocardiographic short term and long term results using precordial mapping. Br Heart J 54:6–10
5. Fioretti P, Brower RW, Lazzeroni E, Simoons ML, Wijns W, Reiber JHC, Bos RJ, Hugenholtz PG (1985) Limitations of a QRS scoring system to assess left ventricular function and prognosis at hospital discharge after myocardial infarction. Br Heart J 53:248–52
6. Herlitz J, Hjalmarson A (1985) The relationship between the electrocardiographically estimated infarct size and 1- and 2-year survival in acute myocardial infarction. Clin Cardiol 8:141–147
7. Palmeri ST, Harrison DG, Cobb FR, Morris KG, Harrell FE, Ideker RE, Selvester RH, Wagner GS (1982) A QRS scoring system for assessing left ventricular function after myocardial infarction. N Engl J Med 306:4–9
8. Schmidt WG, Essen R v, Uebis R, Edelmann B, Hagemann K, Silny J, Rau G (1985) Das Elektrokardiogramm beim akuten Vorderwandinfarkt nach Wiederherstellung der Blutversorgung. Dtsch Med Wschr 110:665–669
9. Vondenbusch B, Offermanns S, Silny J, Essen R v, Schmidt WG, Rau G, Effert S (1984) Präcoordiale EKG-Analyse während Intensivtherapie von Infarktpatienten. Biomed Tech 29 (Suppl):137–138
10. Wagner GS, Freye CJ, Palmeri ST (1982) Evaluation of a QRS scoring system for estimating myocardial infarct size. I. Specificity and observer agreement. Circulation 65:342–347

Author's address:
Dr. W. G. Schmidt
Department of Internal Medicine I
RWTH Aachen
Pauwelsstraße
5100 Aachen
West Germany

Measurement of improvement of left ventricular function after reperfusion using left ventricular angiography

Florence H. Sheehan

Cardiovascular Research and Training Center, University of Washington, Seattle, Washington, 98195 U.S.A.

The efficacy of thrombolytic therapy has been primarily evaluated from the reperfusion rate achieved by the various agents, or from the mortality rate. Since the presumed mechanism by which mortality is reduced by reperfusion is salvage of ventricular function, our studies have measured ventricular function as their endpoint. The studies described in this report were performed in collaboration with Drs. Detlef G. Mathey and Joachim Schofer at Eppendorf University Hospital in Hamburg, West Germany, and Dr. Andras Szente at the Hungarian Institute of Cardiology in Budapest.

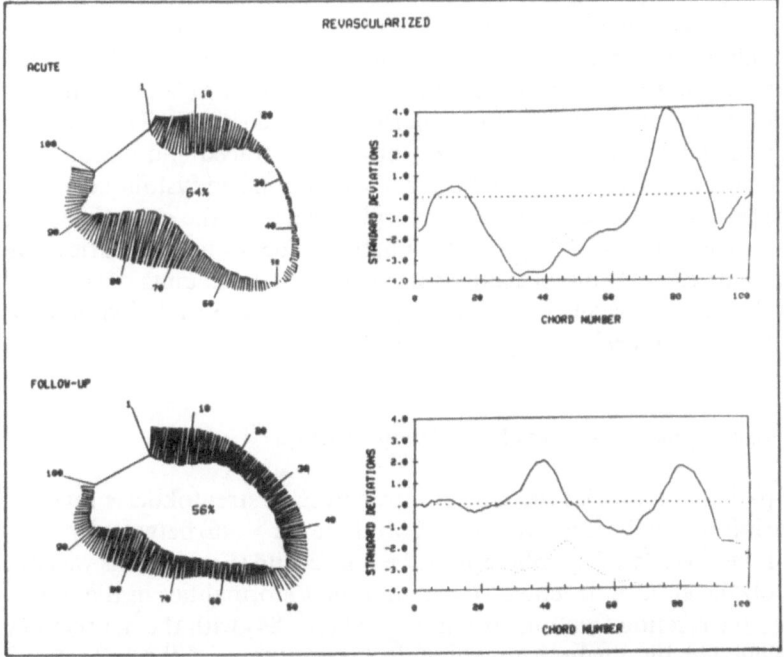

Fig. 1. Patient example. The upper figures display the endocardial contours and wall motion of a patient studied during acute anterior infarction. The lower figures display the same patient's contours and wall motion measured 4 weeks later, following successful reperfusion by intracoronary streptokinase therapy. Despite near normalization of hypokinesis in the infarct region from its acutely depressed value of more than 4 standard deviations below the normal mean, its impact on the ejection fraction was negated by the concomitant decrease in acute compensatory hyperkinesis in the wall opposite the infarction

91

From the beginning of our studies, the disadvantages of measuring only the ejection fraction were apparent. This is demonstrated by the example in Fig. 1. This patient had acute anterior infarction with dyskinesis of the anterior wall, a very severe wall motion abnormality which by our method of analysis is motion more depressed than 3 standard deviations below the normal mean. Reperfusion was achieved with intracoronary streptokinase and on the follow-up angiogram performed about one month later, he had recovery of function in the infarct region. However there was no improvement in the ejection fraction, because he had marked hyperkinesis in the wall opposite the infarct site during acute infarction and this hyperkinesis subsided by the time of follow-up. Thus although there was normalization of motion throughout the ventricle, the ejection fraction did not reflect the improved function because of the opposing changes in the infarct and noninfarct regions. This suggested that the ejection fraction is a relatively insensitive parameter for evaluating the effect of thrombolytic therapy on salvage of myocardial function (8).

Methods for wall motion analysis

The present report describes the data obtained on patients admitted within 3 h after onset of symptoms of myocardial infarction who underwent thrombolytic therapy with intracoronary streptokinase or intravenous urokinase (3, 8). Patients treated with urokinase underwent immediate cardiac catheterization. The cine films of the coronary and ventricular angiograms were sent to the University of Washington for analysis. Wall motion was measured by the centerline method (Fig. 2). The cine ventriculogram is projected and the endocardial contours are traced and digitized. A centerline is constructed midway between the end diastolic and end systolic contours. Motion is measured along 100 chords drawn perpendicular to the centerline, and normalized for heart size (Fig. 2 C). Because the normal value for motion varies with the region of the ventricle, motion measurements are converted to units of standard deviations from the normal mean (Fig. 2 D). Negative values represent hypokinesis and positive values, hyperkinesis (1, 7–9).

Relationship between regional and global ventricular function

Examination of patients studied at the time of intracoronary streptokinase revealed that during acute infarction there is a very poor correlation ($r = .46$) between the ejection fraction and the severity of hypokinesis at the infarct site (Fig. 3). This was due to the influence on the ejection fraction of wall motion abnormalities in the noninfarct region, since the ejection fraction correlated well ($r = .84$) with the net regional abnormality (calculated by algebraically summing the motion of the infarct and noninfarct regions) (10, 11) (Fig. 4).

Similarly there was a very poor correlation between the change in motion in the infarct site and the change in the ejection fraction following thrombolysis (8). For example, in patients who had optimal reperfusion with intracoronary streptokinase and who then underwent bypass surgery there was a very significant improvement in the function of the infarct region (Fig. 5). However, because hyperkinesis in the

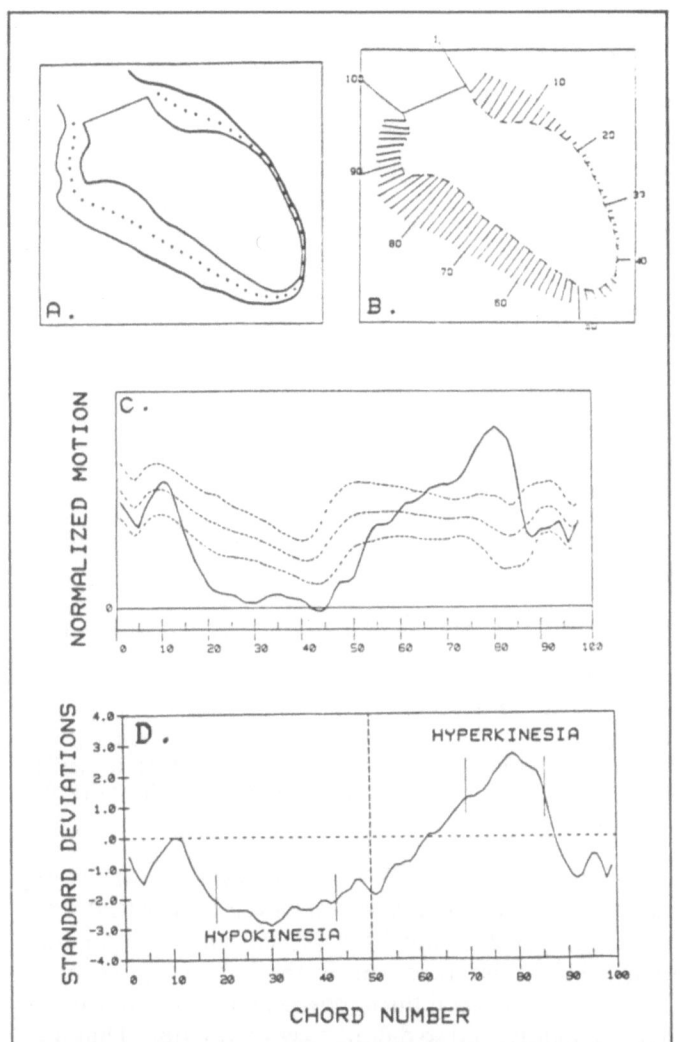

Fig. 2. Centerline method of regional wall motion analysis. **A.** End-diastolic and end-systolic left ventricular endocardial contours and centerline constructed by the computer midway between the two contours. **B.** Motion is measured along 100 chords constructed perpendicular to the centerline. **C.** Motion at each chord is normalized by the end-diastolic perimeter to yield a shortening fraction. Motion along each chord is plotted for the patient (solid line). The mean motion in the normal ventriculogram group (dashed line) and one standard deviation above and below the mean (dotted lines) are shown for comparison. **D.** Standardized motion. The wall motion of the patient is now plotted in units of standard deviations from the normal mean (dotted line). The normal ventriculogram group mean is represented by the horizontal zero line. Vertical lines delimit the most hyperkinetic (HYPER) and most hypokinetic (HYPO) parts of the anterior and inferior regions

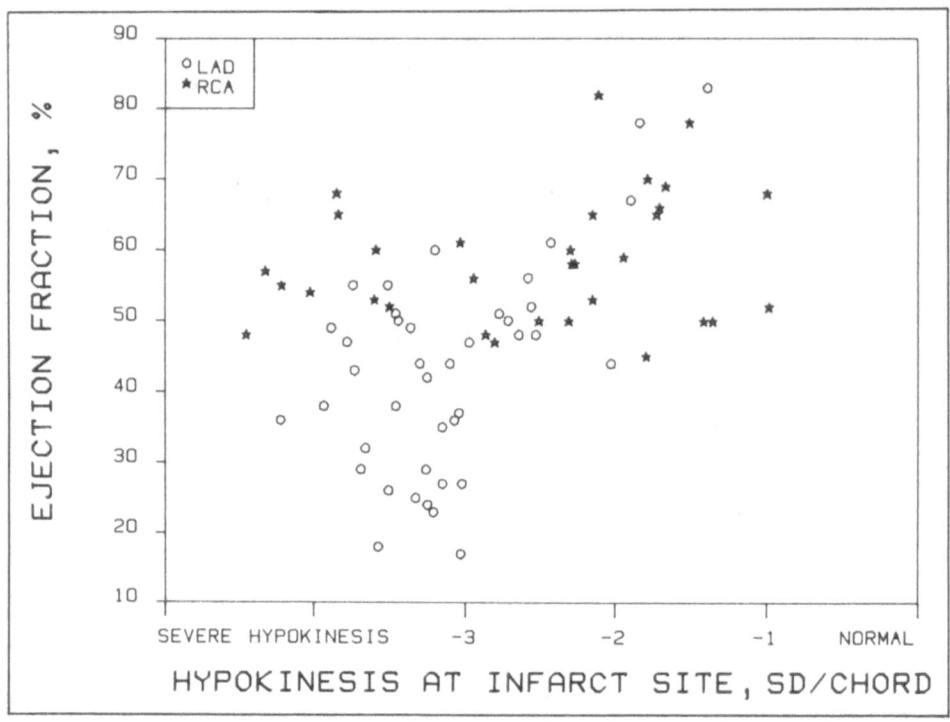

Fig. 3. Ejection fraction plotted against severity of wall motion abnormality in the region of acute myocardial infarction, measured in the most hypokinetic part and expressed in units of standard deviations from normal per chord (SD/chord). [Reprinted with permission from Eur Heart J (11)]

opposite wall decreased between the acute and follow-up studies, there was no significant change in the ejection fraction. In patients who achieved only partial reperfusion, the ejection fraction change reflected actually the decreasing function in the noninfarct region rather than the slight improvement in the infarct region. In patients who never reperfused or who suffered rethrombosis, motion in both infarct and noninfarct regions decreased slightly, and so did the ejection fraction. Thus measurement of wall motion more sensitively reflects the effect of thrombolytic therapy on the function of the infarct region than does the ejection fraction.

Need for biplane ventriculography

One question that has been raised about wall motion analysis, however, is its ability to reflect global function from a single view. Therefore, the data of 67 patients who had biplane ventriculograms in the 30° right anterior oblique (RAO) and 60° left anterior oblique (LAO) views at the time of acute infarction were analyzed (Table 1) (13, 14). In patients who had thrombosis of the left anterior descending coronary artery, hypokinesis in the infarct site was significantly more severe when measured in the RAO projection than in the LAO projection. For patients with right coronary artery (RCA) thrombosis hypokinesis was similar in the two views. Only in the

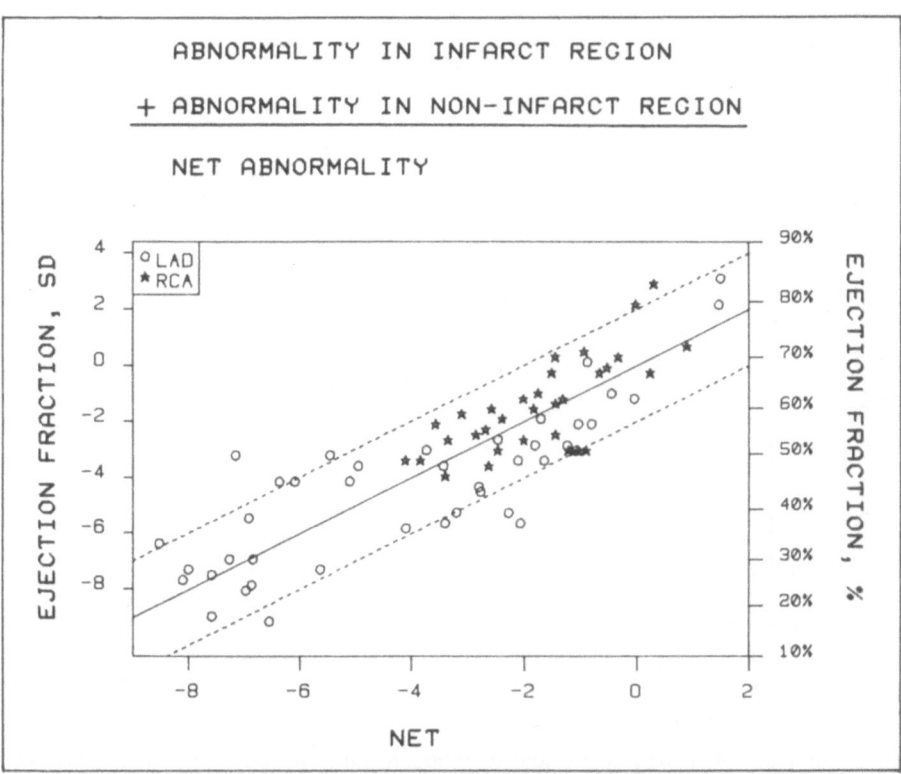

Fig. 4. Ejection fraction plotted against net wall motion abnormality in the infarct and noninfarct regions. Motion is expressed in standard deviations per chord from normal; negative values indicate that motion in the region is depressed and positive values indicate that motion is greater than normal. Symbols indicate patients with anterior (o) and inferior (*) myocardial infarction. [Reprinted with permission from Eur Heart J (11)]

minority of patients with circumflex (CFX) thrombosis was hypokinesis more severe when measured in the LAO projection. This difference was not significant, but the number of patients with CFX thrombosis is small. Thus regional function in infarct patients is more accurately determined from the 30° RAO than from the 60° LAO projection. This indicates that the effect of thrombolytic therapy on function can be evaluated from single plane ventriculograms, except in the small minority of patients with CFX thrombosis, and validates the results of our previous studies.

Factors influencing recovery of ventricular function after reperfusion

The advantage of using quantitative methods to measure sensitive endpoints, such as wall motion in the infarct site, is that it enables identification of factors that influence the recovery of function following reperfusion. For example, significant improvement in wall motion in the infarct region was prevented if there was severe re-

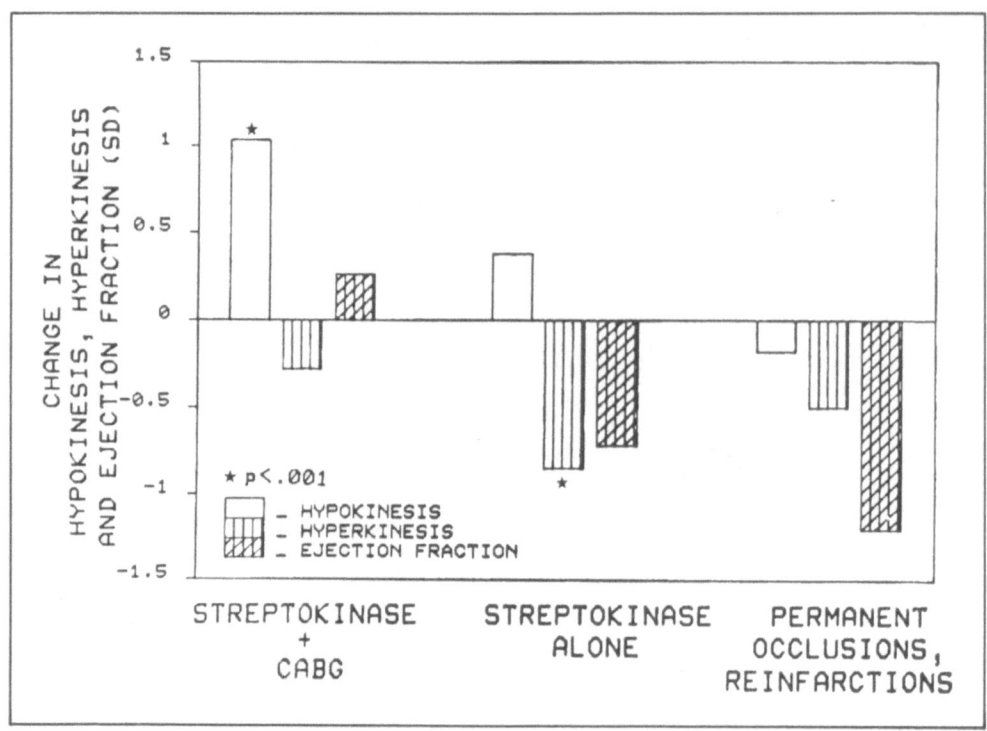

Fig. 5. Change in wall motion in the infarct and noninfarct regions, and in ejection fraction, between acute and follow-up study in patients treated with intracoronary streptokinase. See text for subgroup definition. [Adapted from (8)]

sidual stenosis in the infarct artery following intracoronary thrombolysis, i.e., a minimum diameter less than 0.4 mm, despite angiographic reperfusion (12). However, patients who had a more patent artery following thrombolysis did not all recover, indicating that other factors are also operating.

Another very important factor is the time delay from the onset of symptoms until thrombolysis (3, 4). Patients who were treated within 2 hours after the onset of pain had a significantly greater improvement in wall motion and less residual hypokinesis at the time of follow-up compared to patients who had later treatment. In contrast

Table 1. Biplane analysis of wall motion in the site of acute myocardial infarction

Infarct artery	n	30° RAO	60° LAO	P*
Left anterior descending	36	-3.0 ± 0.9	-2.0 ± 0.8	$< .001$
Right coronary artery	21	-2.2 ± 1.0	-2.1 ± 1.0	$< .001$
Circumflex artery	10	-1.5 ± 1.1	2.2 ± 0.8	NS

Abbreviations: SD = standard deviations from the normal mean, RAO = right anterior oblique, LAO = left anterior oblique.
* Paired t-test

no significant relationship was found between the ejection fraction and either the time delay to treatment or the severity of residual stenosis in the infarct artery.

The change in function in reperfused patients was proportional to the initial abnormality such that greatest improvement was seen in those with severest hypokinesis acutely. This agrees with previous studies reporting that patients with an acute ejection fraction <45% have a greater improvement in function following reperfusion than do patients with more normal function acutely (16). The data essentially indicate that reperfusion results in normalization of ventricular function, but are noteworthy in that patients with akinesis or even dyskinesis have the potential for complete recovery if reperfused.

There was no difference between infarction due to LAD vs. RCA thrombosis in the severity of hypokinesis measured during acute infarction or the magnitude of functional recovery in the infarct region after reperfusion (17).

Clinical implications of improving regional wall motion

The clinical implications of achieving improved regional but not global function are not generally known. However analysis of the relationship between ventricular function measured pre-discharge in reperfused patients and the infarct size as estimated from creatine phosphokinase release curves showed that the severity of hypokinesis in the infarct region correlates well with the infarct size (r = .80), better than did the ejection fraction (r = .72). In addition to its comparatively greater accuracy in indicating infarct size, measurement of regional wall motion may provide a more powerful predictor of survival. This has been reported in four studies comparing wall motion to ejection fraction (Table 2) (2, 18–20). Only in the first study was the centerline method used, which indicates that these results are not method-dependent. Ong et al. (6) disagreed, but used radionuclide ventriculography which has poorer resolution (see below).

Comparison with radionuclide ventriculography

These results and studies by others (17) indicate that measurement of wall motion is important for evaluating myocardial salvage after therapy in infarct patients. It

Table 2. Studies reporting regional wall motion to be a better predictor of survival than ejection fraction

Reference	Reason for catheterization	n	Survival	Type of wall motion analysis
Stadius et al. (18)	Acute MI	227	30 d, 6 mon	Quantitative
Tamaki et al. (19)	Acute MI	108	1–6 yr	Quantitative
Kennedy et al. (2)	Pre-CABG	5024	operative	Qualitative
Weintraub et al. (20)	Diagnosis	411	2 yr	Qualitative

Abbreviations: MI = myocardial infarction, CABG = coronary artery bypass graft surgery.
* In this study, 1 year survival post MI was better predicted by the ejection fraction

would certainly facilitate patient assessment if wall motion could be analyzed using a noninvasive modality such as radionuclide ventriculography. To investigate this possibility, patients enrolled in the NIH Thrombolysis in Myocardial Infarction Trial underwent both contrast ventriculography and radionuclide angiography before discharge. For both imaging modalities the centerline method was used for the wall motion analysis. The results showed that hypokinesis in the infarct site was significantly more severe when measured from contrast ventriculograms than when measured using radionuclide ventriculography (-2.9 ± 0.8 vs. -1.8 ± 0.5 SD/chord, $N = p < .001$) (5). This indicates that wall motion analysis using radionuclide ventriculography has less discriminate power to distinguish infarct patients from normal subjects.

Rest exercise study of ventricular function

Although several reports indicate that the ejection fraction response to exercise predicts survival in patients with chronic coronary artery disease, the accuracy with which this parameter reflects the function of the infarct region in post thrombolysis patients cannot be assumed. Therefore, the rest-to-exercise change in regional and global ventricular function was evaluated in 24 patients studied at least 10 days after thrombolytic therapy. All patients underwent contrast ventriculography at rest and following three minutes of supine bicycle exercise. The rest-to-exercise change in ejection fraction correlated poorly ($r = .38$) with the rest-to-exercise change in wall motion in the infarct site. Reperfused patients could not be distinguished from non-reperfused patients by the ejection fraction response, but the rest-to-exercise change in wall motion in the infarct site was significantly greater in reperfused patients than in the nonreperfused patients, in whom wall motion actually decreased during exercise (15). Thus the exercise ejection fraction response does not always indicate, and cannot be used as a measure of, myocardial salvage in the infarct region in patients who have undergone thrombolytic therapy. Indeed, in almost half of patients with a contrasting exercise response in the anterior and inferior walls (i.e., one wall had increased motion, one wall decreased motion), the ejection fraction response reflected the exercise-induced change in the motion of the noninfarct region.

Summary

In summary, the efficacy of thrombolytic therapy in salvaging myocardial function, and the factors that influence the recovery of function can be sensitively evaluated using regional wall motion analysis. The ejection fraction does not accurately reflect the severity of hypokinesis in the infarct site either at rest or with exercise, due to the influence of hyperkinesis in the noninfarct region. Regional hypokinesis correlates better with infarct size and with survival than does the ejection fraction. However regional hypokinesis is significantly underestimated when measured by radionuclide angiography.

We conclude from these data that for the evaluation of thrombolytic therapy and its ability to salvage myocardial function, regional wall motion analysis should be performed using a high resolution imaging modality.

References

1. Bolson EL, Kliman S, Sheehan F, Dodge HT (1980) Left ventricular segmental wall motion – a new method using local direction information. Comput Cardiol, pp 245–248
2. Kennedy JW, Kaiser GC, Fisher LD, Maynard C, Fritz JK, Myers W, Mudd GM, Ryan TJ, Coggin J (1980) Multivariate discriminant analysis of the clinical and angiographic predictors of operative mortality from the collaborative study in coronary artery surgery (CASS). J Thorac Cardiovasc Surg 80:876–887
3. Mathey DG, Schofer J, Sheehan FH, Becker H, Tilsner V, Dodge HT (1985) Intravenous urokinase in acute myocardial infarction. Am J Cardiol 55:878–882
4. Mathey DG, Sheehan FH, Schofer J, Dodge HT (1985) Time from onset of symptoms to thrombolytic therapy: A major determinant of myocardial salvage in patients with acute transmural infarction. J Am Coll Cardiol 6:518–525
5. McKenzie W, Duncan J, Kayden D, Fetterman R, Greene R, Sheehan F, Bolson E, Dodge H, Canner P, Wackers FJ, Zaret BL (1985) A new method for quantifying regional wall motion on radionuclide angiocardiography (abstr). Circulation 72 (Suppl III): III–480
6. Ong L, Green S, Reiser P, Morrison J (1986) Early prediction of mortality in patients with acute myocardial infarction: A prospective study of clinical and radionuclide risk factors. Am J Cardiol 57:33–38
7. Sheehan FH, Dodge HT, Mathey DG, Brown BG, Bolson EL, Mitten S (1982) Application of the centerline method: Analysis of change in regional left ventricular wall motion in serial studies. IEEE Comput Cardiol, pp 97–100
8. Sheehan FH, Mathey DG, Schofer J, Krebber HJ, Dodge HT (1983) Effect of interventions in salvaging left ventricular function in acute myocardial infarction: A study of intracoronary streptokinase. Am J Cardiol 52:431–438
9. Sheehan FH, Stewart DK, Dodge HT, Mitten S, Bolson EL, Brown BG (1983) Variability in the measurement of regional ventricular wall motion from contrast angiograms. Circulation 68:550–559
10. Sheehan FH, Szente A, Mathey DG, Dodge HT (1984) Discordance between ejection and regional hypokinesis in acute and chronic myocardial infarction (abstr). J Am Coll Cardiol 3:526
11. Sheehan FH, Szente A, Mathey DG, Dodge HT (1985) Assessment of left ventricular function in acute myocardial infarction: The relationship between global ejection fraction and regional wall motion. Eur Heart J (in press)
12. Sheehan FH, Mathey DG, Schofer J, Dodge HT, Bolson EL (1985) Factors determining recovery of left ventricular function following thrombolysis in acute myocardial infarction. Circulation 71:1121–1128
13. Sheehan FH, Schofer J, Mathery DG, Dodge HT, Wygant J, Mitten S, Bolson EL (1985) Comparison of the magnitude of wall motion abnormality visualized in the 30 degree RAO and 60 degree LAO projections. IEEE Comput Cardiol (in press)
14. Sheehan FH, Schofer J, Dodge HT, Wygant J, Mitten S, Bolson EL (1985) RAO vs LAO regional wall motion changes in post-thrombolysis patients (abstr). Circulation 72 (Suppl III):III–22
15. Sheehan FH, Mathey DG, Schofer J, Dodge HT, Mitten S, Bolson EL (1985) Rest-exercise contrast ventriculographic wall motion change post thrombolysis (abstr). Circulation 72 (Suppl III):III–412
16. Smalling RW, Fuentes F, Matthews MW, Freund GC, Hicks CH, Reduto LA, Walker WE, Sterling RP, Gould KL (1983) Sustained improvement in left ventricular function and mortality by intracoronary streptokinase administration during evolving myocardial infarction. Circulation 68:131–138

17. Stack RS, Phillips HR III, Grierson DS, Behar VS, Kong Y, Peter RH, Swain JL, Greenfield JC Jr (1983) Functional improvement of jeopardized myocardium following intracoronary streptokinase infusion in acute myocardial infarction. J Clin Invest 72:34–95
18. Stadius ML, Maynard C, Sheehan FH, Davis K, Fritz JK, Ritchie JL, Kennedy JW (1984) Six month prognosis after acute MI based on clinical and acute angiographic variables from streptokinase trial (WWIST) (abstr). Circulation 70 (Suppl II):II–257
19. Tamaki N, Leinbach RC, McKusick KA (1985) Prognostic importance of changes in regional wall motion in patients with acute myocardial infarction (abstr). Circulation 72 (Suppl III):III–480 III:III–481
20. Weintraub WS, Agarwal JB, Seeclaus PA, McHugh E, BarrAlderfer VA, Helfant RH (1983) Segmental wall motion soore as a predictor of survival in coronary artery disease (abstr). Circulation 68 (Suppl III):III–414

Author's address:

Florence H. Sheehan, M.D.
University of Washington RG-22
Seattle, WA 98195
U.S.A.

Quantitative assessment of regional left ventricular motion after early thrombolysis using endocardial landmarks

P. W. Serruys, H. Suryapranata, C. Slager, F. Vermeer, M. van den Brand, J. Res, F. Verheugt, R. van Domburg, M. Simoons, and P. G. Hugenholtz

Thoraxcenter Rotterdam and the Netherlands Interuniversity Institute

The very existence of several methods (6, 13, 16, 20, 26, 41) to analyze left ventricular wall motion from contrast angiograms indicates that no exact, generally accepted procedure is available to track fixed points along the endocardial wall. In animals, specific sites of the endocardium can easily be followed with endocardially implanted metal clips (5, 32, 44) and roentgen cinematography. For obvious reasons, endocardial markers have not been inserted in humans, although midwall motion (9) and epicardial wall motion (3, 15, 31) have been studied in human hearts with surgically implanted metal markers. However, major differences exist in extent and direction of movements of neighboring endocardial, midwall and epicardial sites as the wall thickens (44, 64). Therefore, none of these methods can provide an accurate description of endocardial wall motion. Recently, we described and evaluated a method to assess left ventricular endocardial wall motion in humans from the pathways of anatomic landmarks recognizable on the endocardial border. For delineation of the endocardial border in the contrast angiogram, an automated high resolution outlining system (60) was employed. In the detected left ventricular contour, small landmarks are available that can be followed throughout the cardiac cycle by analysis of consecutive frames of the cineangiogram. The hypothesis that these landmarks represent specific anatomic sites has been validated by placing minute "harpoons" in the endocardium of piglets. By comparing the mean systolic pathways of these artificial landmarks with those occurring naturally, their usefulness was substantiated.

Subsequently, the naturally occurring landmarks in normal human individuals were determined from left ventricular cineangiograms, and a widely applicable model for the assessment of human left ventricular wall motion was derived.

The applicability of this model is illustrated with use of the results of wall motion analysis in patients with acute myocardial infarction treated by intra-coronary infusion of thrombolytic agents.

To answer the question as to whether thrombolysis is a clinically useful approach in acute myocardial infarction, a randomized trial was started in June 1981. This report details the analysis of the influence of myocardial reperfusion on left ventricular function after attempted recanalization in comparison to similar studies in patients randomly assigned to conventional treatment.

In the randomized trials published thus far, the assessment of global ejection fraction has prevailed (1, 21, 22, 25, 36, 39, 43) since it is relatively easily obtainable. However improvement in global left ventricular function after successful recanalization might be attributed to several factors: salvage of jeopardized myocardium, compensatory hyperactivity of opposite wall segments (42, 54) or changes in pre- and afterload. In

101

an effort to unravel these options, the effect of myocardial reperfusion on left ventricular function has been analysed by measuring systolic regional wall motion.

Methods

Description of the wall motion model

Coordinate system

For quantitative analysis a nonindexed rectangular coordinate system was defined on the basis of the end-diastolic contour. The origin coincides with the end-diastolic apex, the point at maximal distance from the superior aspect of the aortic valve (2). A basal transverse axis, extending from the mitral valve fornix to a point on the opposite anterior wall, was constructed, creating an isosceles triangle with its vertex at the ventricular apex (Fig. 1). The ventricular long axis was defined as the median of this triangle through the vertex; the y axis of the coordinate system coincides with this line.

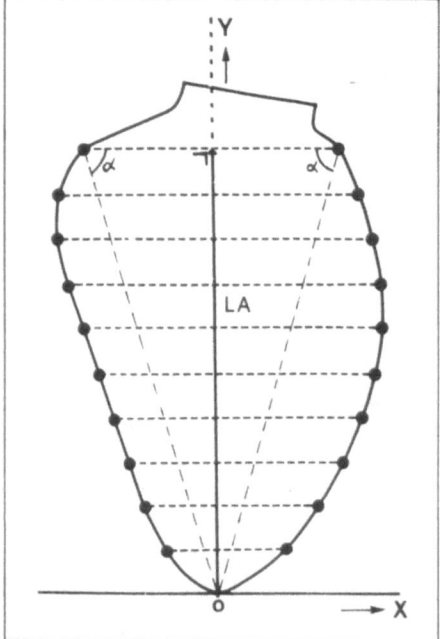

Fig. 1. The median of an isosceles triangle, with its vertex at the ventricular apex and its base extending from the mitral valve fornix, defines the y axis of a rectangular coordinate system. Left ventricular long axis (LA) length is defined as the distance from base to apex. From base to apex a equidistant y levels, 20 end-diastolic starting points are defined for the assessment of pathways of the endocardial landmarks. α = the acute angle; x = x coordinate

102

Normalization

A normalization procedure was carried out to compare the pathways at various endocardial sites of ventricles with different shapes and sizes. First, 10 equidistant points were defined along the long axis. Lines drawn through these points in a direction perpendicular to the long axis defined a total of 20 intersecting points with the end-diastolic contour (Fig. 1). These 20 points were considered to be the initial end-diastolic endocardial sites to be used in assessing the interpolated pathways of the previously mentioned landmarks. For both the human and pig ventricles, left ventricular dimensions were normalized so that for each study group the end-diastolic long-axis lengths became equal to the mean value. As a result of this procedure, corresponding sites had equal y coordinates but still unequal x coordinates. Finally, the normalized systolic trajectories at corresponding sites were shifted parallel to the x axis so that they coincided with the mean value of the individual x coordinates (Fig. 2).

With respect to the coordinate system, the individual pathways were separated into their x and y components, expressed as Δx and Δy. The direction of each pathway was defined as the acute angle (α) between the pathway and the x axis:

$$\alpha = \text{Arc tg} \frac{(\Delta x)}{y}.$$

Endocardial wall motion in pigs

Figure 3 shows the normalized systolic pathways of the endocardial landmarks of each pig (1 a to 8 a) with the systolic pathways of the implanted metal markers of the same ventricles (1 b to 8 b). Comparison of the x and y components of corresponding pathways of endocardial landmarks (Δx_{endo} and Δy_{endo}) and of metal markers

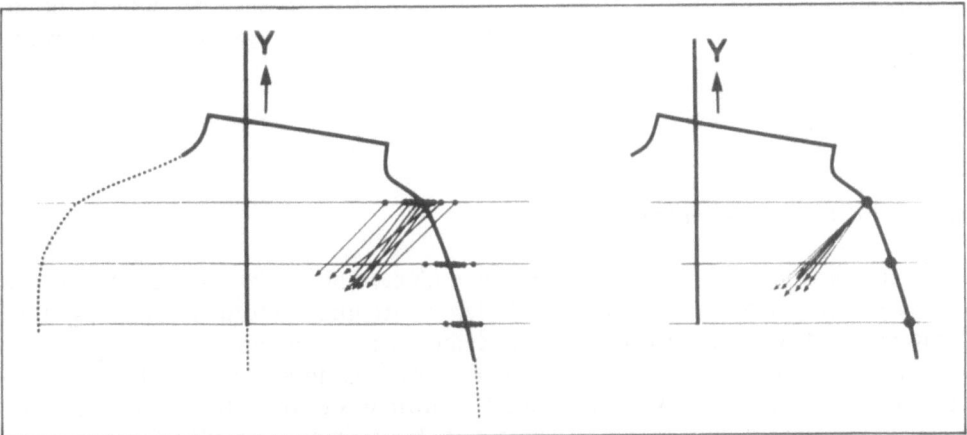

Fig. 2. After normalization of the ventriculograms for long axis length (left), corresponding starting points were shifted along the x axis so that they coincided, resulting in an x coordinate equal to the mean x value (right)

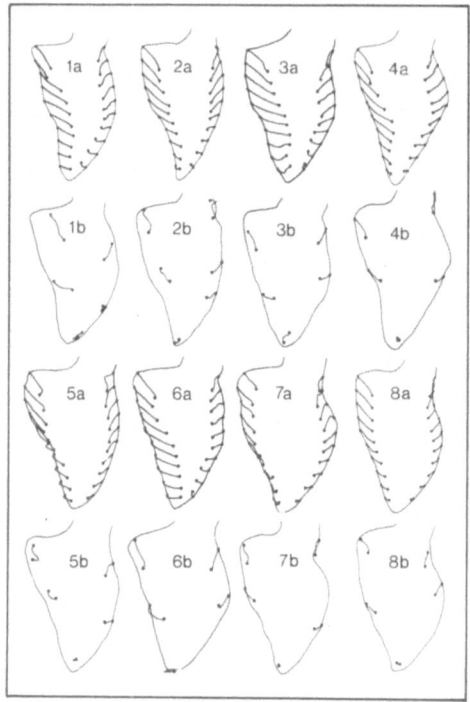

Fig. 3. Normalized left ventricular systolic pathways (1 a to 8 a) of the endocardial landmarks in the eight study pigs are shown with the systolic pathways of the implanted markers (1 b to 8 b) in the same pig ventricles. Note the similarity of the pathways of the landmarks and the markers

(Δx_{metal} and Δy_{metal}) results in a correlation coefficient of 0.74 and 0.86, respectively, with the linear regression equations as follows: $(\Delta x_{endo}) = 0.16$ cm $+ 1.2 \, (\Delta x_{metal})$ and $\Delta y_{endo} = -0.13$ cm $+ \Delta y_{metal}$ (n = 41). The relation between the directions of the endocardial landmark pathways and the metal marker pathways was similarly evaluated:

$$\alpha_{endo} = 0.86 \,_{metal} - 2.9°; \; r = 0.86; \; SEE = 10.3° \; (n = 33).$$

Endocardial wall motion in humans

The coordinates of the 20 sites along the endocardial border were used to define the normalized shape of the end-diastolic left ventricular contour. The mean systolic landmark pathways and their standard deviations are shown in Fig. 4.

The points of intersection of the mean pathways extending from the 10 pairs of opposing end-diastolic sites with the x and y coordinates of the intersection points are depicted of the left side of Fig. 5. The result shown in Fig. 5 can be formulated so that for any point of an end-diastolic contour, the approximate mean direction of motion can be easily calculated. Consider L the length of the end-diastolic long axis as defined in Fig. 1, (x_a, y_a) the coordinates of a point on the anterior wall and $(x_i,$

104

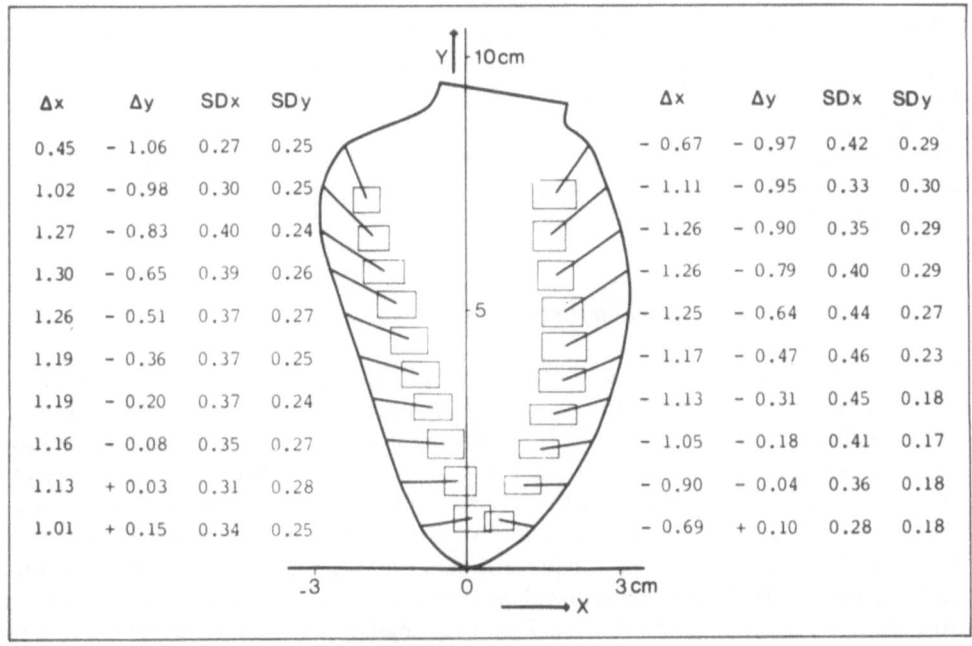

Δx	Δy	SDx	SDy		Δx	Δy	SDx	SDy
0.45	− 1.06	0.27	0.25		− 0.67	− 0.97	0.42	0.29
1.02	− 0.98	0.30	0.25		− 1.11	− 0.95	0.33	0.30
1.27	− 0.83	0.40	0.24		− 1.26	− 0.90	0.35	0.29
1.30	− 0.65	0.39	0.26		− 1.26	− 0.79	0.40	0.29
1.26	− 0.51	0.37	0.27		− 1.25	− 0.64	0.44	0.27
1.19	− 0.36	0.37	0.25		− 1.17	− 0.47	0.46	0.23
1.19	− 0.20	0.37	0.24		− 1.13	− 0.31	0.45	0.18
1.16	− 0.08	0.35	0.27		− 1.05	− 0.18	0.41	0.17
1.13	+ 0.03	0.31	0.28		− 0.90	− 0.04	0.36	0.18
1.01	+ 0.15	0.34	0.25		− 0.69	+ 0.10	0.28	0.18

Fig. 4. Mean systolic left ventricular endocardial landmark pathways in the 23 normal human individuals. The x and y components of each pathway are expressed as Δx and Δy. The rectangles represent the standard deviation (SD) of Δx and Δy

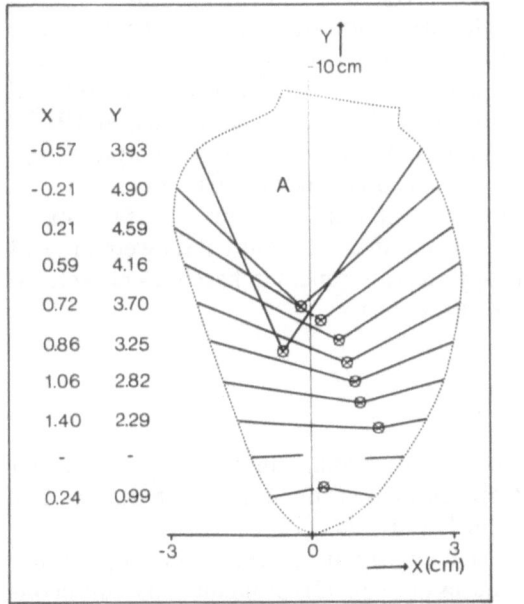

X	Y
-0.57	3.93
-0.21	4.90
0.21	4.59
0.59	4.16
0.72	3.70
0.86	3.25
1.06	2.82
1.40	2.29
-	-
0.24	0.99

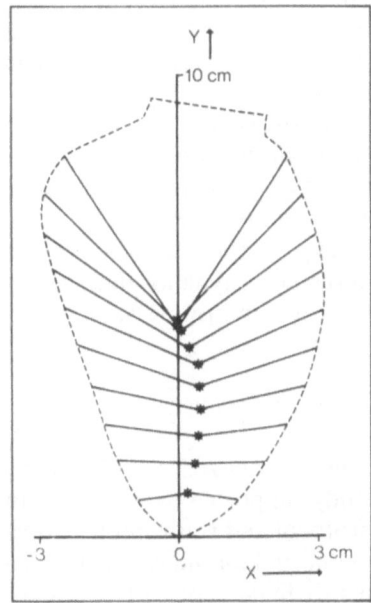

Fig. 5. Points of intersection of the pathways extending from the 10 pairs of opposing starting points (left) and points of intersection of the pathways and direction of regional wall motion using the mathematical expression described in the text (right)

y_i) the coordinates of a point on the opposite inferior wall so that $y_a = y_i = y$. In a first approximation, the coordinates (x_p, y_p) of the point toward which both opposite points will move are then defined by: $x_p = (x_a + x_i)/2$ and $y_p = L(0.57 - 0.53 (1 - 1.1y/L)^{1.4})$.

The difference between corresponding pathway directions on the left and right parts of Fig. 5 is less than 4°, except for the 9.7° difference for the pathway starting from the mitral valve fornix.

Analysis of global and regional left ventricular function

In this trial, global and regional left ventricular function was studied from the 30° right anterior oblique left ventricular cineangiogram. After the end-diastolic and end-systolic frames were determined, stroke volume, global ejection fraction and total cardiax index were computed. In Fig. 6A, examples of the end-diastolic (ED) and end-systolic (ES) contours of the left ventriculogram, as displayed by the analysis system, are shown. Systolic regional wall displacement is determined along a system of 20 coordinates based on the pattern of actual endocardial wall motion in normal individuals (58), and generalized as a mathematical expression amenable to automatic data processing (18, 51). For each segment, segmental volume is computed from the local radius (R) and the height of each segment (1/10 of left ventricular long axis length (L) according to the formula: $1/20\Pi R^2 L$. When normalized for end-diastolic volume, the systolic segmental volume change can be considered as a parameter of regional pump function (Fig. 6 B, C). During systole this parameter expresses quantitatively the contribution of a particular segment to global ejection fraction, termed regional contribution to global ejection fraction or CREF (18). The sum of the values for all 20 segments equals the global ejection fraction. The cross-hatched zones in Fig. 6 D represent the segmental CREF values between the 10th and 90th percentiles, as determined in 20 normal individuals. The segmental CREF values in the anterobasal (segments 1–5), anterolateral (segments 5–9), apical (segments 9, 10, 11 and 12), inferior (segments 12–16) and posterobasal (segments 16–20) wall regions were compared in the control group and in the thrombolysis group.

Data are expressed as mean $\pm$ SD; Paired or unpaired Student t-tests were applied to the hemodynamic data whenever appropriate, differences in baseline characteristics between groups were tested by Fisher's exact test.

Patient selection

This randomized trial of thrombolysis in acute myocardial infarction is a multicenter study supported by the Interuniversity Cardiology Institute in the Netherlands. The protocol and some initial results were published in 1982 (10, 18, 49, 57). These preliminary data indicated that reocclusion of the coronary artery occurred predominantly in patients with severe residual stenoses (14, 46, 52). Immediate percutaneous transluminal coronary angioplasty (PTCA) was therefore added to the procedure in those patients in whom visual inspection of the coronary arteriograms suggested residual stenosis in excess of 60%. When it also became evident that, possibly crucial,

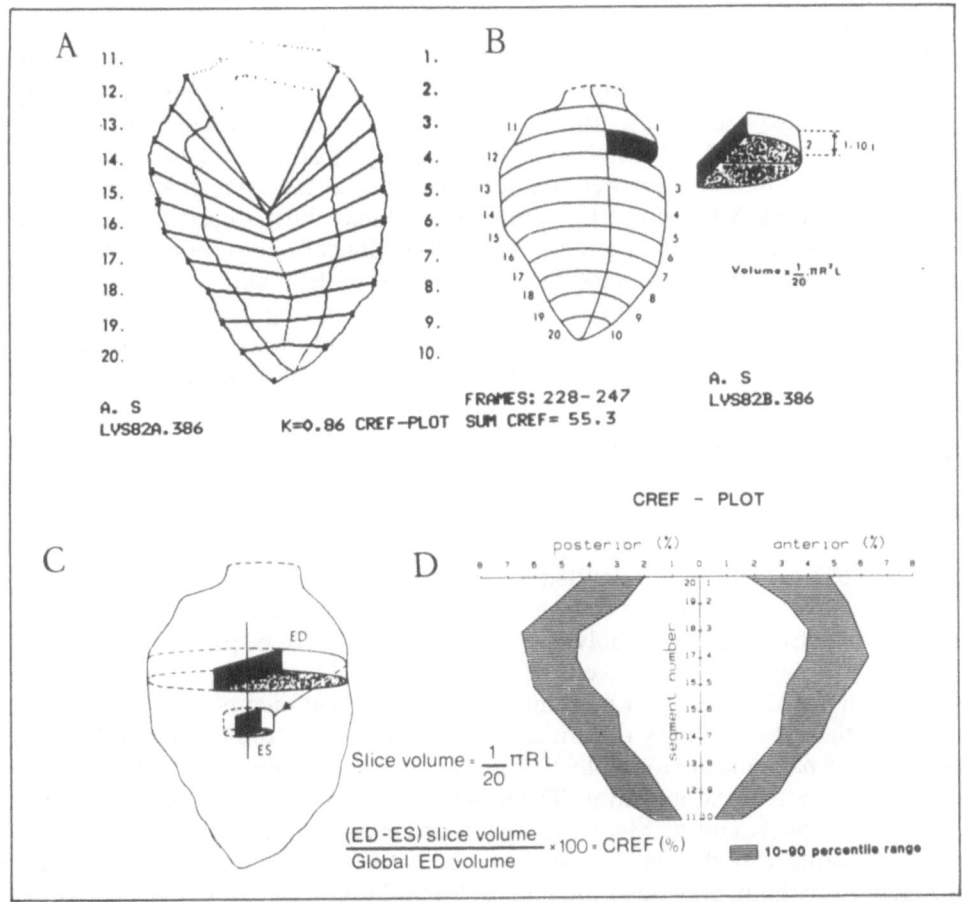

Fig. 6. A. Example of the computer output showing the end-diastolic and end-systolic contours of the 30° RAO left ventriculogram and the system of coordinates along which left ventricular segmental wall displacement is determined. **B.** The left ventricular end-diastolic cavity is divided into twenty half slices. The volume of each half slice is computed according to the given formula, R is radius and L is left ventricular long axis length. **C.** The regional contribution to global ejection fraction (CREF) is determined from the systolic decrease of volume of the half slice which corresponds to a particular wall segment. The systolic volume change is mainly a consequence of the decrease of radius (R) of the half slice. **D.** The shaded zones represent the 10th–90th percentiles area of CREF values in normal individuals. On the X-axis the CREF values of the anterior and infero-posterior wall areas are displayed (%), while on the y-axis the segment numbers of the anterior wall (1–10) and of the infero-posterior wall (11–20) are depicted

time was lost by preparation for catheterization, while other studies (45, 47, 62) reported angiographic confirmation of thrombolysis after intravenous streptokinase, it was decided (January 1984) to give intravenous streptokinase (500,000 U) at the time of admission to the hospital. This meant that thrombolytic therapy was begun approximately one hour before intracoronary streptokinase could be started in this treatment arm. Admission to the study was discontinued in March 1985.

During the study period all patients up to the age of 70 years with chest pain and ECG signs of typical myocardial infarction who were admitted within four hours after the onset of symptoms were eligible for the trial. The usual exclusion criteria for thrombolytic therapy were applied as described in detail in previous reports (10, 18, 57). After inclusion, patients were registered by a central telephone answering service which also provided treatment allocation. Informed consent was obtained from patients allocated to thrombolytic therapy only as proposed by Zelen (66). Patients who refused consent were treated according to the same guidelines as the control group (56). After completion of the streptokinase infusion, complete left and right coronary arteriography was performed. If the clinical condition was stable with left ventricular end-diastolic pressure below 35 mm Hg, left ventriculography in the right anterior oblique projection was done. Coronary arteriography and left ventricular angiography were obtained both in the control group and the thrombolysis-treated group, either before discharge or 4–8 weeks after the acute phase.

Results

Acute and late angiography

A total of 533 patients were admitted to the trial in five participating hospitals; 264 patients were allocated to conventional therapy and 269 patients to thrombolysis. In spite of allocation to thrombolysis angiography could not be performed in 35 patients, as informed consent was refused by 20, while in 3 patients a contraindication occurred or was detected after randomisation, one patient died before angiography and in 6 others the coronary ostium could not be reached from the femoral artery. In the final 5 patients, angiography was not performed as pain and ST elevation resolved shortly after randomization. The results of acute angiography have been summarized in Table 1. Out of 234 patients who underwent acute angiography, 65 had a patent infarct related artery and in 169 this artery was occluded. In 136 patients catheterized without previous intravenous streptokinase, the infarct related vessel

Table 1. Results of acute and late angiography

Acute angiography		Late angiography missing				Late angiography		
		Patient refusal	Death	CABG	Inadequate quality of LV angio.	Other	○	●
264 controls		19	27	4	31	9	90	84
	→ 35 no angiography		4	2	8	2	6	8
269 thrombolysis →	65 ○ → 65 ○	1	1	9	13	5	34	2
	→ 169 ● → 133 ○	11	4	4	17	6	72	19
	→ 36 ●	5	6	5	2	1	10	7
533 patients		41	42	24	71	23	212	120

Patent vessels are indicated (○) and occluded vessels are marked (●); death=patients who died before late angiography was performed; CABG=patients without late angiography due to bypass surgery; other=other missing data e.g. due to transfer to another hospital.

Table 2. Time (minutes) between onset of symptoms and thrombolysis in 127 patients with late angiography.

Range	70–240 min
First quartile	160 min
Median	200 min
Third quartile	255 min

was occluded in 111 (82%) and recanalization was achieved in 88 of these (79%) after 30 minutes (median) of intracoronary infusion of streptokinase. An occluded artery was found in 58 (59%) out of 98 patients who received intravenous streptokinase prior to its intracoronary administration. Subsequently intracoronary streptokinase caused recanalization in 39 patients while in 5 patients the thrombus was perforated by guidewire or angioplasty catheter. Ultimately the infarct related artery remained occluded in 36 out of 234 patients who underwent angiography and at least one attempt at recanalization (15%) while the artery was open at study time or became recanalized in 198 patients (85%). In addition transluminal coronary angioplasty was attempted in 46 patients and was successful in 44 patients. The median time between onset of symptoms and angiographic documentation of a patent infarct related vessel was 200 minutes with a distribution as given in Table 2.

High quality follow-up angiograms were available in 332 patients. These data were missing in 42 patients who died in the intervening period, 24 patients who underwent early bypass surgery, 23 patients who were transferred to another hospital, and 41 patients who refused the second angiogram, while in 71 patients angiograms were made, but were inadequate for quantitative analysis. The angiograms which were available in 332 patients are described in this report. These angiograms were made before discharge in 279 patients (median 11 days) and after discharge in 124 patients (median 42 days). During follow-up angiography patency rates in the control group and thrombolysis group were respectively 52% (90/174) and 77% (122/158) (p = 0.0001). The reocclusion rate in patients recanalized by intracoronary streptokinase was 21% (19 out of 91 patients), while late occlusion in the patients with a patent infarct related vessel at first angiogram was 6% (2 out of 36 patients). Baseline data in Table 3 were comparable in both groups.

Table 3. Baseline data in patients with and without follow-up angiography. The number in each group is given as well as the percentage (%).

	Follow-up angiography		No follow-up angiography	
	Controls	Thrombolysis	Controls	Thrombolysis
n	174	158	90	111
Males	152	130	72	87
Age (mean ± sd)	55 ± 8	55 ± 10	55 ± 9	57 ± 9
Previous infarction	40 (23)	25 (16)	20 (22)	31 (28)
Previous bypass surgery	6 (3)	2 (1)	2 (2)	3 (3)
Anterior wall infarction	69 (40)	79 (50)	47 (52)	51 (46)
Inferior wall infarction	105 (60)	79 (50)	43 (48)	60 (54)

Global left ventricular function: thrombolysis versus conventional treatment

When the hemodynamic data of the control group are compared to those of the thrombolysis group, almost all the parameters listed in Table 4 show significant differences. The global left ventricular ejection fraction in the thrombolysis group was on average 6% (p value = 0.0001) higher than in the control group and this was mainly due to a smaller end-systolic volume in the thrombolysis group (41 ml/m^2 versus 53 ml/m^2 in the control group, p = 0.0004). In addition, the end-diastolic volume was significantly higher and abnormal in the control group compared to the thrombolysis group (95 ml/m^2 vs 84 ml/m^2, p = 0.006) whereas mean aortic pressure and heart rate were not different at the time of the hemodynamic investigation. In Table 5 the hemodynamic data of both groups are shown after exclusion of those 65 patients who had had a previous infarction (40 in the control group and 25 in the thrombolysis group). The differences observed in the entire group (n = 332 patients) between conventional or thrombolytic therapy remain present to a significant degree, but in the thrombolysis group, the ejection fraction is now 6% (p = 0.0002) higher than in the control group while the end-systolic volume is 10 ml/m^2 (p = 0.0015) smaller than in the control group.

Since angiography was not performed in the control group initially, it might be argued that the thrombolysis group had a more favorable outcome due to the higher incidence (28%) of subtotally occluded vessels. Although the randomized approach makes this bias unlikely, we analyzed separately the outcome of patients with the subtotal occlusion and compared it with the results of patients in whom reperfusion of total occlusion was actually achieved during catheterization. The actual beneficial effects of reperfusion in these patients with total occlusion are clearly demonstrated in Table 4; the hemodynamic outcome of these patients did not differ from the outcome of the group with subtotal occlusion.

Global and segmental function in anterior or inferior infarction:
thrombolysis versus conventional treatment

In Table 6 and Fig. 7 the data in patients with inferior infarction are presented. The global ejection fraction shows a 8% difference (p = 0.0001) in favour of the thrombolysis group and this difference in ejection fraction is due to a significantly (p = 0.007) smaller end-systolic volume (37 ml/m^2) when compared to the end-systolic volume of the control group (48 ml/m^2). In Fig. 7 A the regional contribution to ejection fraction values of the patients with inferior infarction assigned to thrombolysis are compared with those assigned to conventional treatment. Depressed regional contribution to ejection fraction was observed in the infero-posterior wall (segments 11–18) as expected, and while regional pump function was significantly better in patients assigned to thrombolysis, it was not normal. In these patients no difference was observed in regional function of the anterior wall. Thus when the recanalization is successful and the infarct related vessel remains patent, there is a significant improvement of function of the inferior wall associated with the subsidence of the initially compensatory augmented functioning of the anterior wall. This latter phenomenon is particularly prominent in the patients who underwent the combined procedure of recanalization and angioplasty (Fig. 7 B) in the acute phase.

Table 4. Left ventricular hemodynamics prior to discharge (n = 332).

	Controls (n = 174)	p value	Thrombolysis (n = 158)	None (n = 14)	○—○ (n = 36)	●—○ (n = 91)	●—● (n = 17)
HR bpm	78 ±15	ns	76 ±13				
Mean AoP mm Hg	88 ±13	ns	90 ±15				
EDP mm Hg	20 ± 9	ns	20 ± 8				
EDV ml/m²	95 ±37	0.006	84 ±33	94 ±33	94 ±42	81 ±30	96 ±46
ESV ml/m²	53 ±31	0.0004	41 ±27	48 ±29	36 ±17	40 ±23	58 ±46
EF %	47 ±14	0.0001	53 ±13	50 ±12	56 ±11	54 ±12	45 ±16
SV ml/m²	42 ±16	ns	43 ±15			p = 0.04	
CI 1/min/m²	3.3± 1.3	ns	3.2± 1.1			p = 0.02	

Values are expressed as means ±SD; Student t-test for unpaired data. Only p values below 0.1 are tabulated. AoP = aortic pressure; CI = cardiac index; EDP = end-diastolic pressure; EDV = end-diastolic volume; EF = ejection fraction; ESV = end-systolic volume; HR = heart rate; SV = stroke volume. None = no acute angiography performed;

○—○ = artery patent at angiography, remained patent;
●—○ = occluded artery recanalized after the intervention;
●—● = occluded artery remained occluded.

Table 5. Left ventricular hemodynamics prior to discharge in patients *without* previous myocardial infarction.

	Controls (n = 134)	Thrombolysis (n = 133)	p value
HR bpm	77 ±13	75 ±13	ns
Mean AoP mm Hg	88 ±13	90 ±15	ns
EDP mm Hg	19 ± 9	19 ± 9	ns
EDV ml/m²	92 ±37	82 ±31	0.03
ESV ml/m²	48 ±29	38 ±22	0.0015
EF %	49 ±13	55 ±12	0.0002
SV ml/m²	43 ±17	44 ±15	ns
CI 1/min/m²	3.3± 1.2	3.3± 1.2	ns

Abbreviations as in Table 4

Table 6. LV hemodynamics in *inferior* infarction prior to discharge.

	Controls (n = 105)	Thrombolysis (n = 79)	p value
HR bpm	77 ±16	74 ±12	ns
Mean AoP mm Hg	88 ±13	91 ±15	ns
EDP mm Hg	19 ± 8	18 ± 8	ns
EDV ml/m²	91 ±35	82 ±32	0.07
ESV ml/m²	48 ±28	37 ±24	0.007
EF %	49 ±13	57 ±11	0.0001
SV ml/m²	43 ±16	44 ±15	ns
CI 1/min/m²	3.3± 1.3	3.3± 1.2	ns

Abbreviations as in Table 4

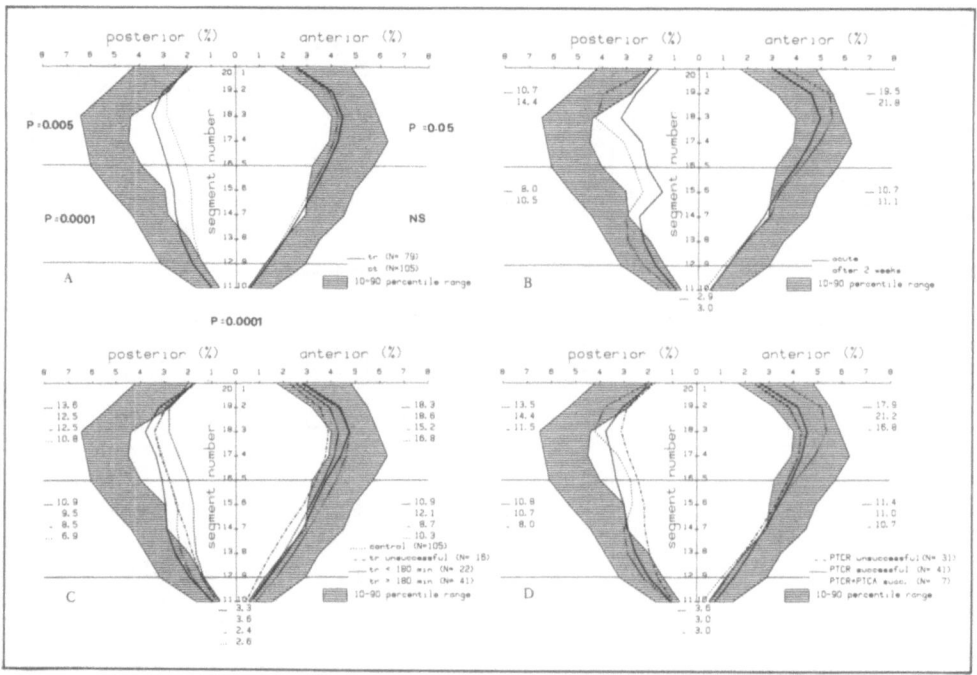

Fig. 7. A. Regional contribution to global ejection fraction (CREF) in 20 segments of the left ventriculogram in patients with inferior infarction. Shaded areas represent the normal range. The regional pump function of the inferior wall (segments 11 to 20) in the thrombolysis treated group (n = 79, solid line) is markedly less depressed than in the conventionally treated group (n = 105, dotted lines). P = p value; ns = non significant. **B.** Change in regional contribution to global ejection fraction from the acute (solid line) to the chronic stage (dotted line) in patients (n = 6) with an inferior infarction who underwent a combined procedure of thrombolysis and angioplasty. **C.** Regional contribution of the inferior wall to global ejection fraction at the chronic stage in the control group and in the thrombolysis group, according to the success of the recanalization at the acute stage and to the time elapsed from the onset of symptoms to treatment. -.-.- control (n = 105), ----- thrombolysis <180 minutes (n = 41), —— thrombolysis >180 minutes (n = 22). **D.** Regional contribution of the inferior wall to global ejection fraction at the chronic stage, in the thrombolysis group (n = 79), according to the initital success and late patency following thrombolysis either with or without angioplasty. -.-.- unsuccessful thrombolysis (n = 31), —— successful thrombolysis (n = 41), ... angioplasty following successful thrombolysis (n = 7)

In Table 7 and Fig. 8, global and regional left ventricular function of patients with anterior myocardial infarction is shown. A significant (p = 0.0025) 7% difference in global ejection fraction is found between both groups due to a smaller end-systolic volume in the thrombolysis group, 45 ml/m² versus 60 ml/m² in the control group (p = 0.006). As Fig. 8 clearly indicates this 7% difference in global ejection fraction in favour of the thrombolysis group is essentially due to a better regional pump function of the anterior wall (segment 1 to 10) and, to a smaller extent, better regional pump function of the infero apical segment (11–15) of the inferior wall (Fig. 8 A). The preceding analysis was based on original treatment allocation, disregarding whether treatment was actually given and whether reperfusion was achieved. The actual effects of reperfusion can better be understood when four subgroups of patients are compared:

Table 7. LV hemodynamics in *anterior* infarction prior to discharge.

	Controls (n = 69)	Thrombolysis (n = 79)	p values
HR bpm	79 ± 13	77 ± 13	ns
Mean AoP mm Hg	87 ± 13	89 ± 14	ns
EDP mm Hg	21 ± 10	21 ± 9	ns
EDV ml/m²	101 ± 39	86 ± 34	0.02
ESV ml/m²	60 ± 34	45 ± 29	0.006
EF %	43 ± 14	50 ± 13	0.0025
SV ml/m²	41 ± 16	42 ± 15	ns
CI l/min/m²	3.2 ± 1.3	3.2 ± 1.1	ns

Abbreviations as in Table 4

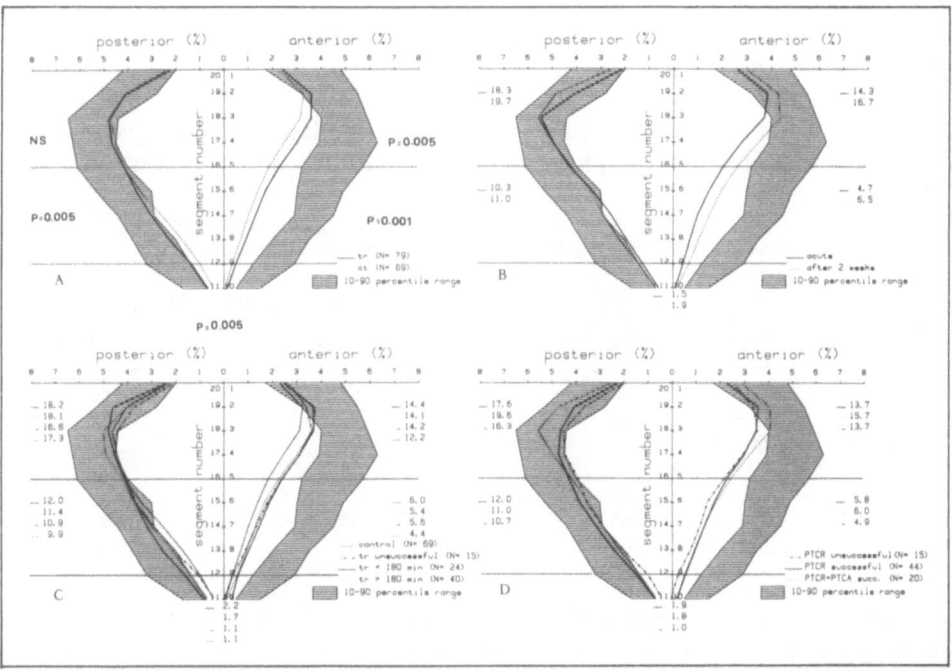

Fig. 8. A. The mean values of regional contribution to ejection fraction in patients with anterior infarction are shown as in Fig. 3. The regional pump function of the antero basal, antero apical, infero apical segments (1–10, 11–15) is significantly better in the thrombolysis group (n = 79, solid line), compared to conventional treatment (n = 69, dotted line). P = p value; ns = non significant. **B.** Change in regional contribution to ejection fraction from the acute (solid line) to the chronic stage (dotted line) in patients (n = 17) with an anterior infarction who underwent a combined procedure of recanalization and angioplasty. **C.** Regional contribution of the anterior wall to global ejection fraction at the chronic stage in the control and in the thrombolysis group, according to the success of the recanalization at the acute stage and to the time elapsed from the onset of symptoms to treatment. -.-.- control (n = 69), ----- thrombolysis <180 minutes (n = 40), —— thrombolysis >180 minutes (n = 24). **D.** Regional contribution of the anterior wall to global ejection fraction at the chronic stage, in the thrombolysis group (n = 79), according to the initial and late patency following success thrombolysis either with or without angioplasty. -.-.- unsuccessful thrombolysis (n = 15), —— successful thrombolysis (n = 44), ... angioplasty following successful thrombolysis (n = 20)

113

a) patients who refused the intervention or who otherwise did not undergo acute angiography; b) patients with either unsuccessful recanalization or late re-occlusion; c) patients with successful recanalization and late patency of the infarct related vessel and d) patients who underwent a successful recanalization, immediately followed by angioplasty. In the patients who could not be recanalized the segmental function of the anterior wall was the worst while the highest preservation of regional function of the anterior wall was observed in these patients who underwent a combined procedure of thrombolysis and angioplasty (Figs. 7 D, 8 D). The magnitude of change in regional function at the infarct site was also related to the time from the onset of chest pain to treatment. Patients treated with thrombolytic therapy within 3 hours had a significantly greater improvement than patients treated later (Figs. 7 C, 8 C). The regional contribution to ejection fraction (CREF) of the infarct zone either anterior or inferior improved by at least 1.5%.

Serial changes in global and segmental function in patients
allocated to thrombolytic therapy

Eighty-two of the patients allocated to thrombolytic therapy had left ventriculograms performed in the acute phase of myocardial infarction and at a follow-up

Table 8. Thrombolysis group: serial LV hemodynamics in *anterior* infarction (n = 38)

	Successful (n = 34)			Unsuccessful (n = 4)		
	Acute	P-value	Chronic	Acute	P-value	Chronic
HR bpm	84 ±13	.007	75 ±14	84 ±16	ns	80 ± 3
Ao mm Hg	82 ±12	.07	85 ± 9	87 ±12	ns	89 ±30
EDP mm Hg	23 ±10	.06	19 ± 8	22 ± 9	ns	26 ± 8
EDV ml/m^2	81 ±32	ns	83 ±27	58 ±22	ns	77 ±11
ESV ml/m^2	42 ±24	ns	41 ±22	28 ± 9	ns	39 ± 4
EF %	49 ±11	.06	53 ±12	50 ± 9	ns	48 ± 7
SV ml/m^2	38 ±14	.04	42 ±13	30 ±15	ns	38 ±10
CI l/min/m^2	3.2± 1.1	ns	3.1± 1.1	2.4± 0.9	ns	3.0± 0.7

Abbreviations as in Table 4. Values are expressed as means ±SD; Student t-test for paired data
Thrombolysis group: serial LV hemodynamics in *inferior* infarction (n = 44)

	Successful (n = 29)			Unsuccessful (n = 15)		
	Acute	P-value	Chronic	Acute	P-value	Chronic
HR bpm	82 ±13	.02	75 ±11	87 ±21	.03	75 ±13
Ao mm Hg	86 ±15	.02	94 ±10	85 ±10	ns	87 ±15
EDP mm Hg	18 ± 8	ns	19 ± 9	20 ±10	ns	19 ± 8
EDV ml/m^2	71 ±22	ns	78 ±29	74 ±27	.0003	93 ±28
ESV ml/m^2	27 ±11	.05	32 ±15	37 ±19	.0006	48 ±26
EF %	61 ± 9	ns	60 ± 8	55 ±10	.004	51 ±11
SV ml/m^2	43 ±16	ns	46 ±16	40 ±15	.08	45 ± 9
CI l/min/m^2	3.6± 1.3	ns	3.5± 1.2	3.4± 1.4	ns	3.3± 0.8

Abbreviations as in Table 4. Values are expressed as means ±SD; Student t-test for paired data

catheterization. In Table 8, the serial changes in global left ventricular function are shown of the patients with anterior and inferior infarction. Following successful recanalization, no significant change in ejection fraction could be demonstrated. In the patients with inferior infarction the improvement of the inferior wall observed between the acute and chronic stage was partially masked by the disappearance of the compensatory actions of the initially enhanced function of the anterior wall (Fig. 7 B). Conversely, when recanalization was unsuccessful a significant deterioration of the global parameters resulted: a decrease of 4% in ejection fraction (p = 0.004), an increase in end-systolic volume from 37 to 48 ml/m^2 (p = 0.0006), and in end-diastolic volume from 74 to 93 ml/m^2 (p = 0.0003). Similar trends were observed in the patients with anterior infarction. In these 82 patients serial changes in regional contribution of the infarct zone to ejection fraction were studied according to the success of thrombolysis either with or without angioplasty (Fig. 9). In the angioplasty group, global ejection fraction increased significantly (p = 0.03) from 51 to 55% from the acute to the chronic stage, an improvement primarily due to a 16% increase in the value of the regional contribution to ejection fraction of the infarct zone.

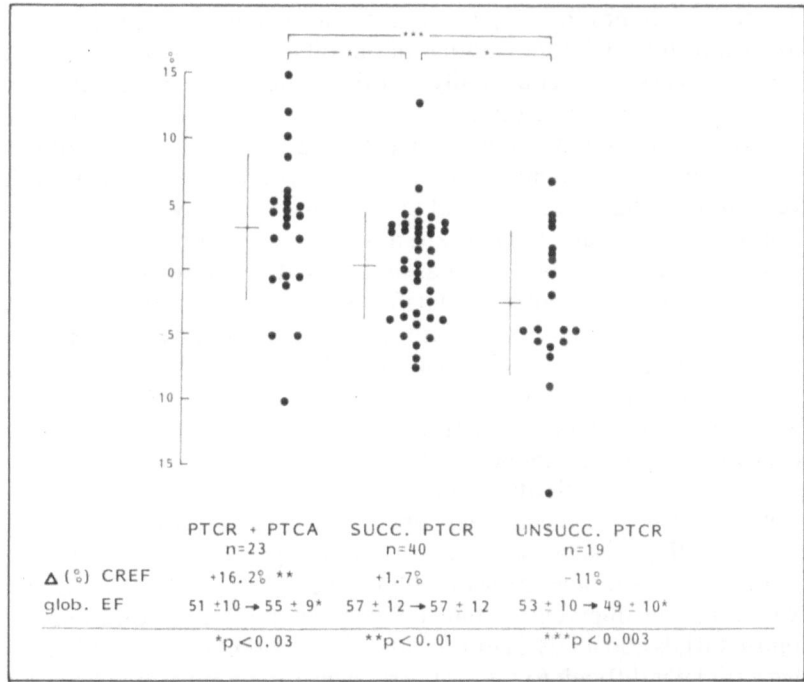

Fig. 9. Changes in regional contribution to global ejection fraction (CREF-IZ, %) of the infarct zone (anterior: segment 1 to 10; inferior: 11 to 20 between the acute phase and the late control. a. Patients either with unsuccessful recanalization or late re-occlusion (unsucc PTCR). b. Patients with successful recanalization and late patency of the infarct related vessel (succ PTCR). c. Patients who underwent a successful recanalization, immediately followed by angioplasty (PTCR + PTCA). abbreviations or symbols: glob. EF = global ejection fraction; Δ = relative increment or decrement; p value < 0.05 are reported (paired or unpaired Student's t-test)

In the group of patients undergoing successful thrombolysis without angioplasty, the global ejection fraction remained unchanged at 57% and was associated with a small increase of 1.7% in the value of the regional contribution to ejection fraction of the infarct zone. Conversely in patients with unsuccessful thrombolysis, the global ejection fraction actually decreased significantly ($p = 0.03$) from 53% to 49%, a change consistent with the 11% decrease in the value of the regional contribution to ejection fraction of the infarct zone.

Discussion

Criticisms of study design

The results of the present study show for the first time in a large randomized multicenter trial that early recanalization of an occluded coronary artery in the acute phase of a myocardial infarction is followed by preservation of global and regional left ventricular function. When compared to the natural fate of the left ventricular function of patients randomly assigned to conventional treatment in most of whom left ventricular function deteriorated, the treated hearts maintained normal end-diastolic and end-systolic volumes thus explaining their normal ejection fraction.

These results are in agreement with the findings of our pilot study (17) where the left ventricular function was assessed sequentially – at the acute and chronic stage – in patients with "successful" or "unsuccessful" recanalization. Similar results have been reported by Rentrop et al. (38), Ganz et al. (11), Mathey et al. (29) and others (9, 40, 48, 61). From these non-randomised studies it appeared that patients with "successful" recanalisation had higher global ejection fractions (by 5–12%) compared to those with "unsuccessful" recanalisation or conventional treatment. Also, it appeared that left ventricular damage was less in those patients who demonstrated spontaneous recanalisation of the infarct related vessel 4–6 weeks after the acute event (9). Schwartz et al. (48) found improvement of the left ventricular function only when recanalisation was achieved within 4 hours. Rentrop et al. (40) suggested that improved left ventricular function after thrombolysis occurred only in patients with collaterals, those with incomplete obstruction before intervention and those in whom complete obstruction was permanently recanalised. Although all these studies have aroused great interest and rekindled enthusiasm for reperfusion, their interpretation is fraught with difficulty as selected patients with successful thrombolysis were compared to patients with persistent occlusions. Such interpretation can carry considerable bias, since patients in whom thrombolysis succeeded are not necessarily similar to those in whom the intervention failed. Such bias can be overcome only by means of randomized trials and analysis of the data on an "intention to treat" basis. However, in such a trial it is difficult to follow the sequence: determination of patient eligibility, coronary arteriography, randomization and attempted reperfusion of patients randomized to special therapy. In this sequence, patients with evolving infarcts who are randomized to conventional therapy would be obliged to undergo emergency coronary arteriography without sufficient potential benefit to outweigh the attendant risk. To overcome this difficulty we randomized all patients who were eligible on clinical grounds but obtained consent for performing coronary arteriography only from those assigned to reperfusion therapy. This procedure has been proposed by Zelen (66) for the comparison of a new method of treatment with an accepted mode of therapy. Since angiography was not performed in the control group initially, radionuclide angiography was carried out at the bedside on the first or second day after admission and repeated before hospital discharge in the control group as well as in the thrombolysis group. The results indicate no change in global left ventricular ejection fraction between the second day and hospital discharge in the control group. In thrombolysis patients left ventricular ejection fraction before discharge was 3.7% higher than during the first measurement. Accordingly left ventricular ejection fraction after 10 to 20 days was approximately 4% higher when thrombolysis was compared with conventional treatment. This difference was significant in the whole group, in patients treated with intracoronary thrombolysis only, in patients with a first infarction and in both anterior and inferior infarction. In fact, the beneficial effects of thrombolysis in the currently reported trial gain great significance as infarct size, ventricular function and survival all were significantly improved on the "intention to treat" principle applied to consecutive patients.

Current results of randomized trials

The results of the five reported but smaller randomized trials with intracoronary streptokinase (21, 22, 25, 36, 39) conflict with the data presented here. Khaja et al. (22) found that intracoronary streptokinase was more effective than placebo (intracoronary infusion of dextrose) in achieving reperfusion, but they detected no difference in left ventricular function at 12 days and at 5 months. Kennedy et al. (21), Leiboff et al. (25) and Raizner et al. (36) also demonstrated no difference in the radionuclide ejection fraction at discharge in patients with anterior or inferior myocardial infarction treated with intracoronary streptokinase or controls, although they achieved reperfusion and decreased mortality. In all these studies the intervention was instituted much later than in the current one. The median interval between the onset of symptoms and angiographic documentation of a patent infarct related vessel in the present study was 200 minutes while the other two major trials, included patients up to 12 hours after the onset of symptoms. In the study of Khaja et al. (22) and Raizner et al. (36) the time period between chest pain and onset of infusion of streptokinase was 5.4 and 5.6 hours respectively, in the Western Washington Trial the mean time until randomization and the start of streptokinase infusion was 276 minutes (21, 43), while Rentrop started intracoronary streptokinase on average 350 minutes after the onset of symptoms (39). The shorter delay achieved in our study is also reflected by the higher recanalization rate (79%) compared to the Western Washington Trial (68%). The differences between this and the only other large (250 pts.) randomized trial may be crucial, since they confirm experimental data that recovery of ischemic myocardium cannot be achieved after four hours of coronary occlusion (23). Since in some patients recurrent episodes of occlusion alternating with spontaneous reperfusion may occur (8), it remains possible that the salutary effect of thrombolysis in such patients extends beyond a time interval of 4 hours. However such beneficial influences are completely outweighed by the inability to achieve recovery of functions and tissue in the majority of patients and the increased chance of reperfusion injury as ischemic time lengthens. Schwartz et al. (48) clearly demonstrated no benefit from late reperfusion (4 hours) which is in agreement with all animal experiments (27, 35, 37). He (48), Anderson et al. (1) and our data agree in demonstrating streptokinase to have a major beneficial effect on the left ventricular function provided it is given within 4 hours after onset of symptoms.

The magnitude of change in regional function in the infarct zone was also significantly influenced by the time elapsed between the onset of chest pain and the actual recanalization. Patients with an infarct related vessel recanalized within 3 hours had significantly greater improvement than patients treated later. The regional contribution to ejection fraction (CREF) of the infarct zone improved by at least 1.5% in patients treated within 3 hours with either anterior of inferior infarction. As recently demonstrated by Mathey et al. (30) thrombolysis should be administered within 2 hours after the onset of symptoms to obtain maximal recovery of ventricular function.

The inclusion of mechanical perforation and transluminal coronary angioplasty as part of the recanalization procedure and the introduction of intravenous administration of streptokinase in the second treatment arm prior to the cardiac catheterization provide another major difference with previously reported studies. Transluminal coronary angioplasty was employed in two of the five hospitals who had extensive experience with this procedure. It was carried out when residual obstruction was considered 60% or more after thrombolysis (14, 52) in order to prevent reocclusion. Patients so treated had a lower mortality and a lower incidence of reinfarction than patients successfully treated with streptokinase alone. Although these results may be biased by the selection of patients with lesions suitable for transluminal coronary angioplasty, hemodynamically stable after thrombolysis, these findings are in agreement with earlier observations that the recovery of regional left ventricular function is greatest in patients with a minimal residual stenosis after the intervention (53, 54). Experimental studies have also shown that restriction of flow during reperfusion results in relative underperfusion of, and continued ischemia in, the subendocardium (24).

Analysis of global and regional wall motion

Measurement of the global ejection fraction is a rather crude method which may not detect improvement of regional left ventricular function. Therefore analysis of left ventricular wall motion in the infarction area at risk which potentially should benefit most from reperfusion, must be carried out in order to detect any real effect of reperfusion (12, 54, 63). In fact, increased motion of the non-infarcted regions of the heart, often kept the global ejection fraction within normal limits despite severe regional hypokinesia in the infarction area. Contractile performance of the non-infarcted area may be enhanced by the Frank-Starling mechanism and by increased levels of circulating catecholamines in the first hours. After subsidence of compensatory augmented motion in the non-infarction regions of the heart, which masked significant deterioration in regional wall motion, initially maintained global left ventricular function declined. Here, again, regional wall motion must be measured to adequately assess this effect. Significant improvement of regional function in the "infarct zone" was observed in inferior as well as in anterior locations although significant changes in regional function of the remote "non infarct zone" occurred at the acute as well as at the chronic stage.

The analysis of regional left ventricular function was based on automated, high resolution, frame to frame edge detection of left ventricular contour. This system allows fast and reliable acquisition of single left ventricular contour, every 20 msec, all over a complete cardiac cycle (58, 60). Many wall motion models have been proposed to approximate actual endocardial motion, which reflects the problems investigators had to establish a geometric framework upon which to judge whether the motion of the endocardial contour is normal or abnormal (4). All these methods assess wall motion in terms of extent of shortening at specific points on an axis reference system, although it is highly unlikely that a particular endocardial site coincides with one of these axes during the entire cardiac cycle. The wall motion analysis system we used is based on the motion pattern of small irregularities at the left ventricular endocardial border (endocardial landmarks) which can be detected in the contrast cineangiogram with the above mentioned automated endocardial outlining system (58, 60). This endocardial landmark pathway has been tested previously in 23 normal human left ventricles and validated in pigs with metal endocardial markers inserted with a percutaneous, retrograde, transvascular approach (18, 59). This wall motion analysis is unaffected from the translation and rotation of the heart, thus permitting an actual study of the segmental wall motion and derived parameters.

Early after myocardial infarction, the uninvolved portion of the heart is generally thought to maintain function and metabolism, unless coexisting stenoses of additional vessels cause ischemia of the non infarcted segments (34). Yet, after experimental myocardial infarction, the clearly non ischemic portions of the heart muscle also show changes in energy metabolism and a decline in norepinephrine content (28, 65). Other investigators have reported decreased lactate extraction and ischemic histologic changes, like swelling of mitochondria or reduction in tissue glycogen content, in areas of myocardium remote from the site of coronary occlusion. However, when the infarcted area is reperfused early, the decline in contractility of non infarcted heart muscle appears to be reversible, limited to the early post-infarction (7) period (10 days). Other data, during and after open heart surgery indicate that a longer delay up to 4 weeks might be needed to achieve a full recovery (50). This overall improvement in the ischemic areas and the high (85%) patency of the infarct related artery after the intervention as well as other aspects of the design of this study, show the major significance of early recanalization in order to achieve the goal of preservation of left ventricular function. The results of the present study also indicate that reperfusion may need to be supplemented by additional revascularization procedures such as angioplasty in order to optimize the changes of obtaining full functional recovery. Its beneficial effects evident in this large series of patients studied over an extended time period, might explain the observed reduction (from 16% to 9%) in one year mortality (55).

Prognostic implications

The Multicenter postinfarction research group (33) reported that patients with higher global ejection fraction had better one year survival after myocardial infarc-

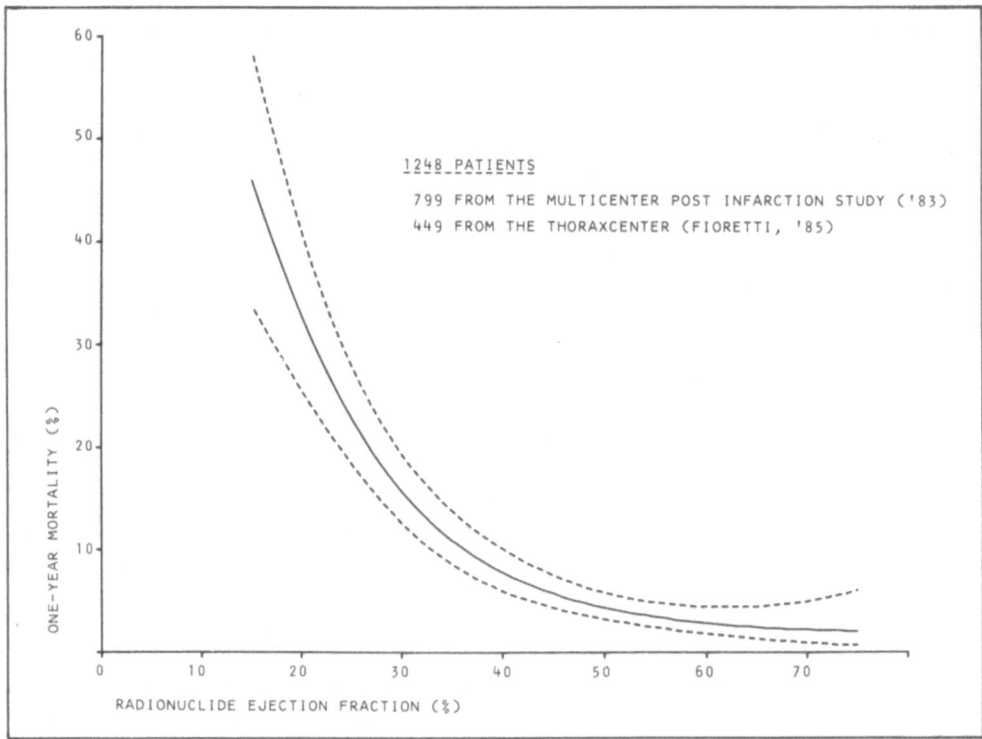

Fig. 10. One-year mortality as a function of radionuclide ejection fraction (%) measured at hospital discharge after acute myocardial infarction. The solid line between the dashed lines indicates the corresponding 95% confidence interval. The calculations are based on pooled data from the Multicenter Post Infarction Study (33) and the Thoraxcenter (P. Fioretti, personal communication, 1985)

tion, independent of the extent of coronary disease. Similar data were found in a follow-up study of 449 hospital survivors at the Thoraxcenter (Fioretti P., personal communication, 1985). Pooling the results of these studies, a curvilinear relationship between the one year mortality rate and global ejection fraction can be constructed (Fig. 10). When the currently observed improvement of left ventricular ejection fraction from 47% in controls versus 53% in patients allocated to thrombolysis is interpreted in this manner, the one year mortality should indeed be reduced from approximately 16% to 12% after thrombolysis, a projection which corresponds to our observations. Thus, the explanation for the reduced mortality must in the main be ascribed to the restoration of left ventricular function, rather than by any other mechanism.

References

1. Anderson JL, Marshall HW, Bray BE et al (1983) A randomized trial of intracoronary streptokinase in the treatment of acute myocardial infarction. N Engl J Med 308:1312–1318
2. Brower RW (1980) Evaluation of patient recognition rules for the apex of the heart. Cath Cardiovasc Diagn 6:145–157

3. Brower RW, Katen HJ ten, Meester GT (1978) Direct method for determining regional myocardial shortening after bypass surgery from a radiopaque markers in man (1978). Am J Cardiol 41:1222–1229
4. Brower RW, Meester GT (1976) Computer based methods for quantifying regional left ventricular wall motion from cine ventriculogram. Comp in Card 55–62
5. Carlsson E, Milne ENC (1967) Permanent implantation of endocardial tantalum screws. A new technique for functional studies of the heart in the experimental animal. J Can Assoc Radiol 19:304–309
6. Chaitman BR, Bristow JD, Rahimtoola SH (1973) Left ventricular wall motion assessed by using fixed external reference systems. Circulation 48:1043–1054
7. Corday E, Kaplan L, Meerbaum S, Brasch J, Constantini C, Lang TW, Gold H, Rubins S, Osher J (1975) Consequence of coronary arterial occlusion on remote myocardium: effects of occlusion and reperfusion. Am J Cardiol 36:385–393
8. Davies GJ, Chierchia S, Maseri A (1984) Prevention of myocardial infarction by very early treatment with intracoronary streptokinase. N Engl J Med 311:1488–1492
9. de Feyter PJ, Van Eenige MJ, van der Wall EE et al (1983) Effects of spontaneous and streptokinase-induced recanalisation on left ventricular function after myocardial infarction. Circulation 67:1039–1044
10. Fioretti P, Simoons ML, Serruys PW, van den Brand M, Fels PW, Hugenholtz PG (1982) Clinical course after attempted thrombolysis in myocardial infarction. Result of pilot studies and preliminary data from a randomized trial. Eur Heart J 3:422–432
11. Ganz W, Buchbinder N, Marcus H, Mondkar A, Maddahi J, Charuzi Y, O'Connor L, Shell W, Fischbein MC, Kass R, Miyamoto A, Swan HJC (1981) Intracoronary thrombolysis in evolving myocardial infarction. Am Heart J 101:4–13
12. Gribier A, Berland J, Champond O, Moore N, Behar P, Letac B (1983) Intracoronary thrombolysis in evolving myocardial infarction. Sequential angiographic analysis of left ventricular performance. Br Heart J 50:401–410
13. Harris LD, Clayton PD, Marshall HW, Warner HR (1974) A technique for the detection of asynergistic motion of left ventricle. Comput Biomed Res 7:380–394
14. Harrison DG, Ferguson DW, Collins SM, Skorton DJ, Eriksen EE, Kioschos JM, Marcus ML, White CW (1984) Rethrombosis after reperfusion with streptokinase: Importance of geometry of residual lesions. Circulation 69:991–999
15. Harrison DC, Goldblatt A, Braunwald E, Glick G, Mason DT (1963) Studies on cardiac dimensions in intact, unanaesthetized man. I. Description of their techniques and their validation. Circ Res 13:448–467
16. Herman MV, Heinle RA, Klein MD, Gorlin R (1967) Localized disorders in myocardial contraction. N Engl J Med 227:222–232
17. Hooghoudt TEH, Serruys PW, Reiber JHC, Slager CJ, van den Brand M, Hugenholtz PG (1982) The effects of recanalization of the occluded coronary artery in acute myocardial infarction on left ventricular function. Eur Heart J 3:416–421
18. Hooghoudt TEH, Slager CJ, Reiber JHC, Serruys PW, Schuurbiers JCH, Meester GT, Hugenholtz PG (1980) "Regional contribution to global ejection fraction" used to assess the applicability of a new wall motion model in patients with asynergy. Comput Cardiol IEEE Comput Soc: 253–256
19. Ingels NB, Daughters GT, Stinson EB, Alderman EL (1975) Measurement of midwall myocardial dynamics in intact man by radiography of surgically implanted markers. Circulation 52:859–867
20. Ingels NB, Mead CW, Daughters GT, Stinson EB, Alderman EL (1978) A new method for assessment of left ventricular wall motion. In: Computers in Cardiology. IEEE Computer Society, Long Beach, CA, pp 57–61
21. Kennedy JW, Ritchie JL, Davis KB, Fritz JK (1983) Western Washington randomized trial of intracoronary streptokinase in acute myocardial infarction. N Eng J Med 309:1477–1482
22. Khaja F, Walton JA, Breymer JF, Lo E, Osterberger L, O'Neill WW, Colfer HT, Weiss R, Lee T, Kurian T, Goldber AD, Pitt B, Goldstein S (1983) Intracoronary fibrinolytic therapy in acute myocardial infarction. Report of a prospective randomized trial. N Engl J Med 308:1305–1311
23. Laffel GL, Braunwald E (1984) Thrombolytic therapy: a new strategy for the treatment of acute myocardial infarction. N Engl J Med 311:710–717

24. Lang TW, Corday E, Gold H, Meerbaum S, Rubins S, Constantini C, Hirose S, Osher J, Rosen V (1974) Consequences of reperfusion after coronary occlusion: Effects on hemodynamic and regional myocardial metabolic function. Am J Cardiol 33:69–81

25. Leiboff RH, Katz RJ, Wasserman AG, Bren CB, Schwartz H, Varghese J, Ross AM (1984) A randomized, angiographically controlled trial of intracoronary streptokinase in acute myocardial infarction. Am J Cardiol 53:404–407

26. Leighton RF, Wilt SM, Lewis RP (1974) Detection of hypokinesis by quantitative analysis of left ventricular cineangiograms. Circulation 50:121–127

27. Maroko PR, Libby P, Ginks WR, Bloor CM, Shell WE, Sobel BE, Ross J Jr (1972) Coronary artery reperfusion. I. Early effects on local myocardial function and the extent of myocardial necrosis. J Clin Invest 51:2710–2716

28. Mathes P, Romig D, Sack D, Erhardt W (1976) Experimental myocardial infarction in the cat. I. Reversible decline in contractility of noninfarcted muscle. Cir Res 38:540–546

29. Mathey DG, Kuck KH, Tilsner V, Krebber HT, Bleifeld W (1981) Non-surgical coronary artery recanalization in acute transmural myocardial infarction. Circulation 63:489–497

30. Mathey DG, Sheehan FH, Schofer J, Dodge HT (1985) Time from onset of symptoms to thrombolytic therapy: A major determinant of myocardial salvage in patients with acute transmural infarction. JACC 6:518–525

31. McDonald JG (1970) The shape and movements of the human left ventricle during systole. Am J Cardiol 26:221–230

32. Mitchell JH, Wildenthal K, Mullins CB (1969) Geometrical studies of the left ventricle utilizing biplane cine-fluorography. Fed Proc 28:1334–1343

33. Multicenter Postinfarction Research Group (1983) Risk stratification after myocardial infarction. N Engl J Med 50:266–272

34. Naccarella FF, Weintraub WS, Agarual JB, Helfant RH (1984) Evaluation of "Ischemia at a distance": effect of coronary occlusion on a remote area of left ventricle. Am J Cardiol 54:869–874

35. Pairolero P, Hallermann FJ, Ellis F Jr (1970) Left ventriculogram in experimental myocardial infarction. Radiology 95:311–316

36. Raizner AE, Tortoledo FA, Verani MS, Reet van RE (1985) Intracoronary thrombolytic therapy in acute myocardial infarction: a prospective, randomized controlled trial. Am J Cardiol 55:301–308

37. Reimer KA, Lowe JE, Rasmussen MM, Jennings RB (1977) The wavefront phenomenon of ischemic cell-death. 1. Myocardial infarct size vs duration of coronary occlusion in dogs. Circulation 56:786–794

38. Rentrop KP, Blanke H, Karsch KR (1982) Effects of nonsurgical coronary reperfusion on the left ventricle in human subjects compared with conventional treatment. Am J Cardiol 49:1–8

39. Rentrop KP, Feit F, Blanke H, Stecy P, Schneider R, Rey M, Horowitz S, Goldman M, Karsch K, Meilman H, Cohen M, Siegel S, Sanger J, Slater J, Gorlin R, Fox A, Fagerstrom R, Calhoun WF (1984) Effects of intracoronary streptokinase and intracoronary nitroglycerin infusion on coronary angiographic patterns and mortality in patients with acute myocardial infarction. N Engl J Med 311:1457–1463

40. Rentrop P, Smith H, Painter L, Holt J (1983) Changes in left ventricular ejection fraction after intracoronary thrombolytic therapy. Results of the Registry of the European Society of Cardiology. Circulation 68 (Suppl 1):55–66

41. Rickards A, Seabra-Gomes R, Thurstone P (1977) The assessment of regional abnormalities of the left ventricle by angiography. Eur J Cardiol 5:167–182

42. Rigaud M, Rocha P, Boschat J, Farcot JC, Bardet J, Bourdarias JP (1979) Regional left ventricular function assessed by contrast angiography in acute myocardial infarction. Circulation 60:130–139

43. Ritchie JL, Davis KB, Williams DL, Caldwell J, Kennedy JW (1984) Global and regional left ventricular function and tomographic radionuclide perfusion: The Western Washington intracoronary streptokinase in myocardial infarction trial. Circulation 70 (Suppl 5):867–875

44. Rushmer RF, Crystal DK, Wagner C (1953) The functional anatomy of ventricular contraction. Circ Res 1:162–170

45. Schröder R, Biamino G, Leitner ERV, Brüggeman T, Heitz J, Vöhringer HF, Wegscheider K (1983) Intravenous short-term infusion of streptokinase in acute myocardial infarction. Circulation 67:536–548
46. Schröder R, Vöhringer H, Linderer T, Biamino G, Brüggemann T, Leitner ERV (1985) Follow-up after coronary arterial reperfusion with intravenous streptokinase in relation to residual myocardial infarct artery narrowings. Am J cardiol 55:313–317
47. Schwartz F, Hofmann M, Schuler G, von Olshausen K, Zimmermann R, Kübler W (1984) Thrombolysis in acute myocardial infarction: effect of intravenous followed by intracoronary streptokinase application on estimates of infarct size. Am J Cardiol 53:1505–1510
48. Schwartz F, Schuler G, Katus H, Hofmann M, Manthey J, Tilmanns H, Mehmel HC, Kübler W (1982) Intracoronary thrombolysis in acute myocardial infarction: duration of ischemia as a major determinant of late results after recanalisation. Am J Cardiol 50:933–937
49. Serruys PW, Brand M van den, Hooghoudt TEM, Simoons ML, Fioretti P, Ruiter J, Fels PhW, Hugenholtz PG (1982) Coronary recanalization in acute myocardial infarction: immediate results and potential risks. Eur Heart J 3:404–415
50. Serruys PW, Brower RW, ten Katen HJ, Meester GT (1980) Recovery from circulatory depression after coronary artery surgery. Eur Surg Res 12:369–382
51. Serruys PW, Wijns W, van den Brand M, Meij S, Slager C, Schuurbiers JCH, Hugenholtz PG, Brower RW (1984) Left ventricular performance regional blood flow, wall motion and lactate metabolism during transluminal angioplasty. Circulation 70:25–36
52. Serruys PW, Wijns W, van den Brand M, Ribeire V, Fioretti P, Simoons ML, Kooijman CJ, Reiber JHC, Hugenholtz PG (1983) Is transluminal coronary angioplasty mandatory after successful thrombolysis? Quantitative coronary angiographic study. Br Heart J 50:257–265
53. Sheehan FH, Mathey DG, Schofer J, Dodge HT, Bolson EL (1985) Factors determining recovery of left ventricular function following thrombolysis in acute myocardial infarction. Circulation 71:1121–1128
54. Sheehan FH, Mathey DG, Schofer J, Krebber HJ, Dodge HT (1983) Effect of interventions in salvaging left ventricular function in acute myocardial infarction: a study of intracoronary streptokinase. Am J Cardiol 52:431–438
55. Simoons ML, Serruys PW, Brand van den M, Baer F, de Zwaan C, Res J, Verheugt FWA, Krauss XH, Remme WJ, Vermeer F, Lubsen J (1985) Improved survival after early thrombolysis in acute myocardial infarction: a randomized trial conducted by the Interuniversity Cardiology Institute in the Netherlands. Lancet i:578–582
56. Simoons ML, Serruys PW, Fioretti P, van den Brand M, Hugenholtz PG (1983) Practical guidelines for treatment with beta-blockers and nitrates in patients with acute myocardial infarction. Eur Heart J 4:129–135
57. Simoons ML, Wijns W, Balakumaran K, Serruys PW, Brand van den M, Fioretti P, Reiber JHC, Lie P, Hugenholtz PG (1982) The effect of intracoronary thrombolysis with streptokinase on myocardial thallium distribution and left ventricular function assessed by blood-pool scintigraphy. Eur Heart J 3:433–440
58. Slager CJ, Hooghoudt TEH, Reiber JHC, Schuurbiers JCH, Booman F, Meester GT (1979) Left ventricular contour segmentation from anatomical landmark trajectories and its application to wall motion analysis. Comput Cardiol IEEE Comput Soc: 347–350
59. Slager CJ, Hooghoudt TEH, Serruys PW, Schuurbiers JHC, Reiber JHC, Meester GT, Verdouw PD, Hugenholtz PG (1985) Quantitative assessment of regional left ventricular motion using endocardial landmarks. JACC (in press)
60. Slager CJ, Reiber JHC, Schuurbiers JCH, Meester GT (1978) Contouromat: a hardwired left ventricular angioprocessing system. I. Design and application. Comput Biomed Res 11:491–502
61. Smalling RW, Fuentes F, Matthews MW, Freund GC, Hicks CH, Reduto LA, Walker WE, Sterling RP, Gould KL (1983) Sustained improvement in left ventricular function and mortality by intracoronary streptokinase administration during evolving myocardial infarction. Circulation 68:131–138
62. Spann JF, Sherry S, Carabello BA, Maurer AH, Cooper EM (1984) Coronary thrombolysis by intravenous streptokinase in acute myocardial infarction: acute follow-up studies. Am J Cardiol 53:655–661

63. Stack RS, Phillips HR, Grierson DS, Behar VS, Kong Y, Peter RH, Swain JL, Greenfield IC (1983) Functional improvement of jeopardized myocardium following intracoronary strep-tokinase infusion in acute myocardial infarction. J Clin Invest 72:84–95

64. Wildenthal K, Mitchell JH (1969) Dimensional analysis of the left ventricle in unanaesthetized dogs. J Appl Physiol 27:115–119

65. Wyatt HL, Forrester JS, da Luz P, Diamond GA, Chagrasulis R, Swan HJC (1976) Functional abnormalities in nonoccluded regions of myocardium after experimental coronary occlusion. Am J Cardiol 37:367–372

66. Zelen M (1979) A new design for randomized clinical trials. N Engl J Med 300:1242–1245

Authors' address:

P. W. Serruys, M.D.
Thoraxcenter
Erasmus University
Catheterization Laboratory
Postbus 1738
3000 DR Rotterdam
The Netherlands

Positron emission tomography of the heart

U. Büll

Abteilung Nuklearmedizin, Aachen (F.R.G.)

Myocardial ECT methods, PET and SPECT provide information on the three-dimensional distribution of radionuclides within the myocardium. Potassium analogues or fatty acids may be used with either method. With PET, however, physiological tracers such as oxygen, ammonium, carboxides and labelled glucose may be exclusively employed. Moreover, with PET, adequate correction for photo-attenuation and depth-independent resolution yield quantitative information on tracer concentration in vivo. Thus, PET enables clinicians to look beyond blood flow and cardiac function to probe the biochemistry of the heart. The radionuclides employed are shown in Table 1. There are three types of radiopharmaceuticals; one labels the blood pool, the second labels the blood flow, and the third is employed to measure myocardial metabolism.

From Schelbert's work (4) we know that measurements of myocardial blood flow in vitro by the microsphere method correlate very well with the MBF in vivo if we use the ultrasound correction of the wall thickness in this special case (Fig. 1). And the PET infarct size measured by Sobel and Meyer (5) as early as 1979 by the 11-Carbon labelled palmitate method gave a good correlation between morphological infarct size and the CPK activity depletion and between morphological size and the PET infarct size (Fig. 2).

From these basic investigations we can conclude that myocardial PET is reliable in coronary artery disease. As Fig. 3 shows, ammonium and palmitic acid revealed low flow and low metabolism within the same area of ischemia. We can thus say that regional myocardial blood flow measured by PET correlates very well with tissue sample counting. And PET estimates of infarct size are in good agreement with post-

Table 1. Positron-emitting radiopharmaceuticals for the study of the heart with PCT [From (4)]

(a) Blood pool imaging agents
^{11}CO and $C^{15}O$ (bound to haemoglobin in red blood cells)

(b) Indicators of myocardial blood flow
^{68}Ga- or ^{62}Cu-labelled albumin microspheres
^{38}K, ^{82}Rb
[^{15}O]-water
[^{13}N]-ammonia

(c) Tracers of myocardial metabolism
[^{11}C]-palmitic acid
[^{11}C]-acetic acid
[^{18}F]-2-deoxy-2-fluoro-glucose, [^{11}C]-2-deoxyglucose
^{13}N and ^{11}C amino acids
[^{11}C]-pyruvic acid, [^{11}C]-lactic acid

125

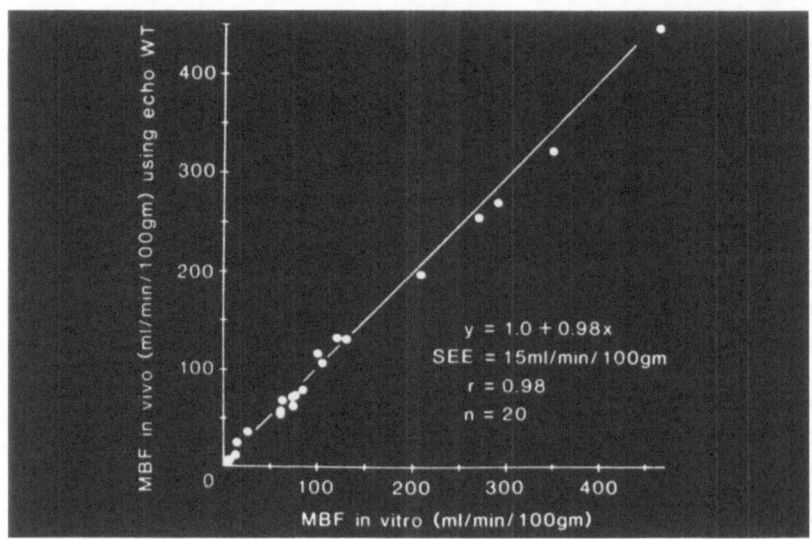

Fig. 1. Regional myocardial blood flow (MBF) measured in vivo with PET (^{68}Ga microspheres and arterial reference sample) vs. tissue sample counting. Ultrasound wall thickness determination (echo WT) was used for WT correction. [From (4)]

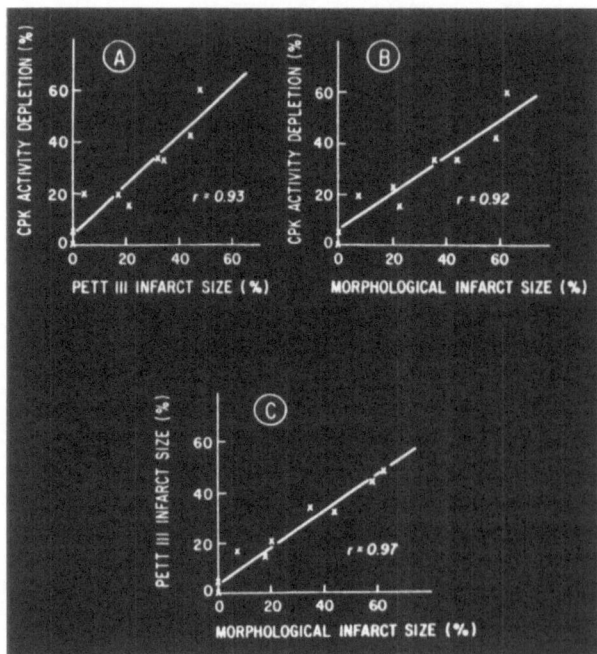

Fig. 2. Correlation between myocardial creatinin phosphokinase (CPK) depletion and PET estimates of infarct size with fatty acids in canine hearts (A) or morphological infarct size (B).[From (5), courtesy of M. S. Klein]

126

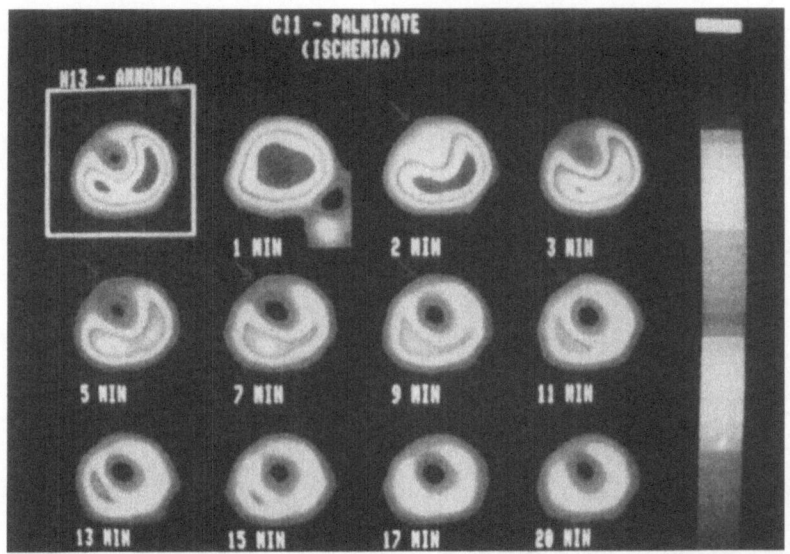

Fig. 3. Perfusion (^{13}N) and fatty acid (FFA) metabolism (1–20 min after injection) during pacing-induced ischemia with PET. Note similar reduction of flow and metabolism in the ischemic region (arrow). [From (4)]

mortem measurements. Thus PET is a reliable method for measuring myocardial perfusion in coronary artery disease.

Schelbert demonstrated that in low flow areas, if the myocardium is still viable but is compromised, it switches from fatty acid metabolism to glycolysis. And thus, one may image the metabolism of 18-F-labelled glucose within an area of low flow and distinguish the perfused myocardium (white) from the nonperfused but still viable myocardium (red) (Fig. 4).

As shown in Table 2, a group working in Liège under De Landsheere (1) presented a paper on a group of 25 patients with MI, 15 treated with intravenous streptokinase and 9 with conventional therapy. They transduced Schelbert's work into a ratio. They found the glucose-to-flow ratio (G:F) in the heart to be normal at 1.4. If the ratio is higher, then the flow measured by 38-K is low and the glucose uptake is high. In the patient shown in Fig. 5, the ratio is 2.90 by low flow. One can see (Table 2) that the high ratios are found only in the group after thrombolysis. They are not found in the group of patients under conventional therapy, where glucose metabolism and blood flow decrease simultaneously. The 'early group' in this table indicates that the patients were examined 10 ± 4 days after the ictus. In the cases with non-transmural infarction, and only in these cases, the ratio increased in the group treated with conventional therapy. The Liège group conclude that patients with compromised, but still viable, myocardium documented by these high ratios may benefit from surgery or even from dilation.

Turning now to the title of this session, limitations, costs, and risks, PET application is mainly limited by costs for cyclotron, the machine, and the team. The total costs per year according to Evens (2) (from the Mallinckrodt Institute in St. Louis) amount to US$ 585 000 ($ 292/hour) for the production of radionuclides and chemis-

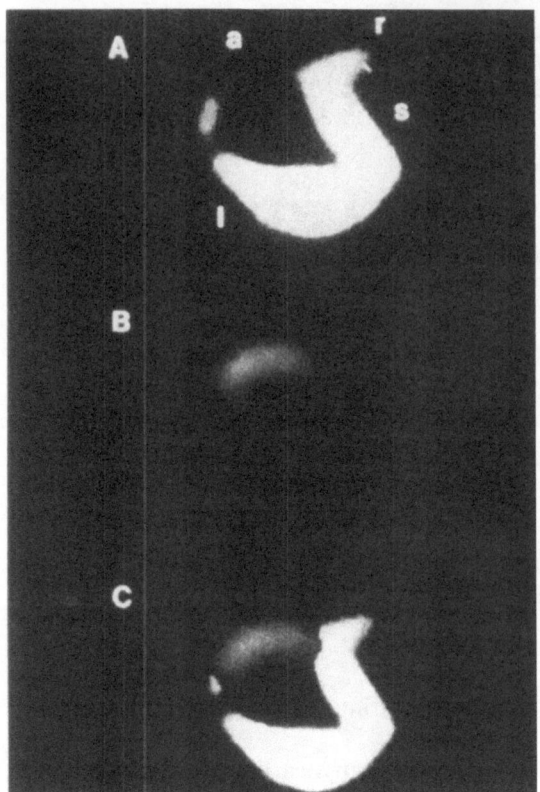

Fig. 4. Perfusion (A) and glucose uptake (B) in an infarcted area. Note decreased perfusion in still metabolic active tissue. [From (4)]

try, while the imaging unit costs $ 644 000 ($ 322/hour). The price per examination at 500 examinations per year is more than $ 1000, and at 2500 examinations it is $ 353. But this means 50 patients per week, which is a high rate. We have no risks, we have a low radiation burden, we have non-invasive application.

In the future we hope that PET costs would be reduced. Using generator systems to replace the very expensive cyclotron would bring costs down. We already have two systems, the 68-Germanium 68-Gallium and the 82-Strontium-82-Rubidium generator, yielding radionuclides for PET to label red blood cells. Or we can apply the PET capacities to double-head gamma cameras which are now routinely used in nuclear medicine laboratories. Further, we can aim at replacing PET by SPECT, but

Table 2. High G:F (glucose-to-flow) ratios in the infarcted area ("early" group). Courtesy of De Landsheere (1)

	Anterior MI		Inferior MI		Non transmural MI	
	N	Mean G:F	N	Mean G:F	N	G:F
15 THR. T	8/10	2.36 ± 0.44	5/5	2.30 ± 0.21	0/0	–
Conv. T	0/5	–	0/1	–	1/3	2.02

THR. T = thrombolytic therapy

128

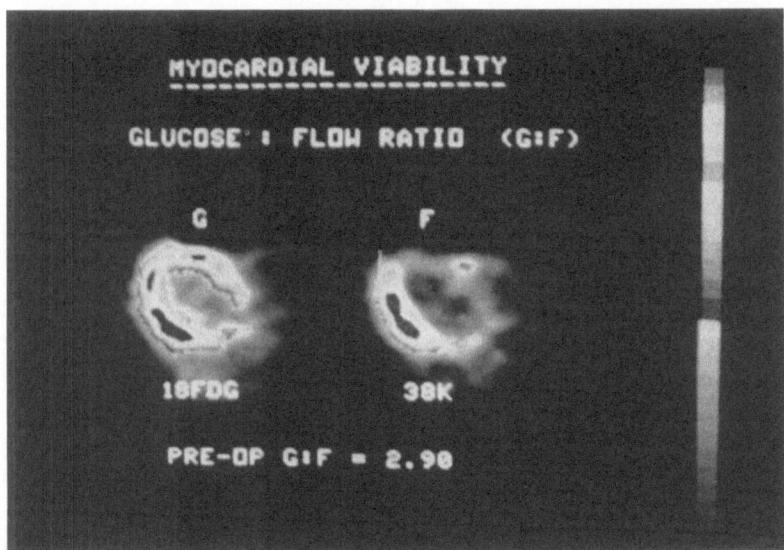

Fig. 5. Ratios of glucose-to-flow (G:F) by PET, employing ^{18}F-desoxyglucose and ^{38}K as markers in a patient with AMI treated by thrombolysis. The ratio of 2.9 indicates viable (but less perfused) myocardium. [From (1), courtesy of De Landsheere]

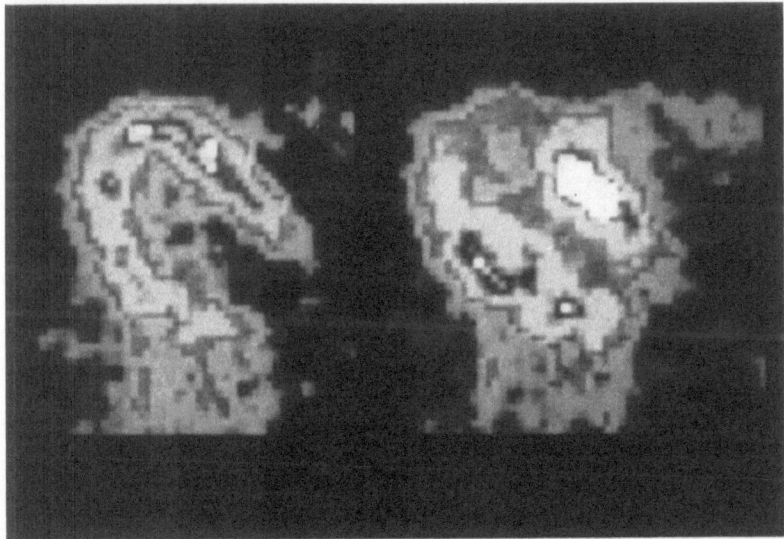

Fig. 6. Transient ischemia, illustrated by ^{82}Rb (from a generator) and PET. Normal flow at rest (left). After exercise (with dipyridamole and handgrip), a perfusion defect occurred (right). [From (3), courtesy of L. Gould]

that is in the even more distant future. At the moment for SPECT, we already employ labelled myocardial blood flow agents (99m Tc-BIN), that represents a new group of substances, and 123-I-labelled fatty acid. What we do not have yet is a method for absolute quantification, and we cannot use glucose metabolism and physiological tracers with these two types of replacements.

But I would like to draw your attention finally, to results obtained with the Strontium-Rubidium generator. Lance Gould (3) works in Houston with a Rubidium generator in addition to a PET machine. Figure 6 shows a patient of his with a coronary stenosis at rest (left) and after dipyridamole combined with hand grip-exercise. The perfusion increases in normal areas, but not in the compromised area beyond the stenosis. Gould thus found a regional ratio (exercise-to-rest) of coronary flow less than 3 in such areas, and this ratio gave a very high sensitivity (21/22 (95%)).

In conclusion, I would like to quote a remark made by Heinz Schelbert at an imaging conference in Washington recently: "Currently PET can be used to diagnose end-stage CAD. In the future, however, PET may detect the disease much earlier, and the catastrophic end result may be prevented by intervening in the disease process at the biochemical level."

References

1. De Landsheere C et al. (1985) Viable ischemic myocardium after an acute infarction: demonstration at rest using combined study of flow and glucose uptake; influence of thrombolytic therapy. Eur Congr Nucl Med, London, Sept 1985
2. Evens RG et al. (1983) Cost analysis of positron emission tomography for clinical use. Am J Roentgenol 141:1073
3. Gould KL et al. (1985) Clinical feasibility, sensitivity and specificity of positron cardiac imaging without a cyclotron using generator produced Rb-82 for the diagnosis of CAD. Eur Congr Nucl Med, London, Sept 1985
4. Schelbert HR (1982) The heart. In: Ell PJ, Holman BL (eds) Computed Emission Tomography. Oxford University Press, p 91ff
5. Klein MS, Sobel BE (1979) Fatty acid uptake and metabolic imaging of the heart. In: Willarson JT (ed) Nuclear Cardiology. FA Davis, Philadelphia, p 165

Author's address:
Prof. Dr. U. Büll
Abteilung Nuklearmedizin
Medizinische Fakultät der RWTH
Klinikum Aachen
Pauwelstraße 1
5100 Aachen
West Germany

Discussion

KÜBLER:

I would like to warn against a too extensive interpretation of metabolic data obtained by positron emission computer tomography. For instance, if glucose or glucose derivatives are used to indicate viability of the myocardium, this is always based on the hypothesis that a maintained glycolytic pathway is identical with myocardial viability. There are certain experimental conditions however, in which this is not the case: if you look at the energy metabolism of the myocardium in the post-ischemic area, the first thing which deteriorates is the mitochondrial function, and there is an enhanced glycolytic flux despite marked deterioration of myocardial metabolism. A second word of warning concerns flow interpretation, even if ammonium is taken as a marker. Ammonium is a very good flow marker under normal conditions, but with ischemia, involving a pH change, ammonium is no longer a good indicator of myocardial flow because its uptake in the myocardial cell not only depends afterwards on the trapping reaction, but also on the N-ion exchange ratio, which in itself is pH dependent. The values are therefore greatly changed during ischemia.

Question:

Does PET enable us to determine if myocardium is stunned and will recover its function, or if myocardium is irreversibly damaged by ischemia?

BÜLL:

Yes, data indicate that this is probable, but we have no final confirmation.

HUGENHOLTZ:

This is not very satisfactory, as it is vitally important for clinicians to know whether these techniques really do have a future. Clinicians need to know if it is worthwhile to initiate a new technique. For us it is absolutely vital to know the boundary between the salvageable and the unsalvageable cell by a non-invasive method. Will this promise of a non-invasive technique, at present expensive but perhaps cheaper later be fulfilled, or do you think it is a dead-end?

BÜLL:

No, it is by no means a dead-end. Our only problem at the moment is the lack of money to establish a unit like this, and there are only a few centres in the world which deal with the heart. Mainly they deal with the brain. There is a centre in Liège and another in Los Angeles, and there are plans in Germany and the Netherlands to establish PET centres for both brain and heart. We will then be able to collect enough data to draw firm conclusions.

Planar and tomographic scintigraphic studies in connection with coronary thrombolysis

D. G. Mathey and J. Schofer

Department of Cardiology, University Hospital Eppendorf, Hamburg (West Germany)

Reinfarction in the first days after successful thrombolysis occurs in 10 to 20% of patients (1, 2). Percutaneous transluminal coronary angioplasty (3) or bypass surgery (4) have been shown to prevent reinfarction in selected patients (3, 4). Because of a certain risk involved, these methods should only be applied in those patients in whom a clinically relevant limitation of infarct size could be achieved. Therefore, myocardial salavage should be assessed immediately after thrombolysis.

1. Intracoronary 201-thallium scintigraphy before and after thrombolysis

In patients undergoing intracoronary thrombolysis the assessment of myocardial salvage is possible by means of intracoronary myocardial scintigraphy with thallium-201 (5). Because of excessively high background activity after repeat intravenous thallium injections, which would be necessary before and after thrombolysis, the intracoronary route of administration is preferable to obtain high quality, background-free scintigrams (Fig. 1, upper panel). An intravenous study in the same patient shows marked extracardiac activity in the gastrointestinal tract even after one thallium injection, which makes it impossible to visualize the inferior defect clearly seen after intracoronary injection (Fig. 1, lower panel).

Ideally, a thallium defect present prior to reperfusion will disappear completely after re-opening of the infarct artery and thallium re-injection into the reopened vessel (Fig. 2). In a second group of patients, thallium uptake after thrombolysis may only be seen in the border zone of the infarct. An irreversible defect in the center of the infarct persists. In a third group, the initial thallium defect will remain unchanged despite thallium re-injection into the re-opened infarct artery.

It is not yet known whether new thallium uptake after reperfusion indeed reflects viable myocardium. We addressed this question by comparing new thallium uptake after thrombolysis with the change in wall motion in the infarct area. We found that wall motion improved significantly more in patients with complete thallium uptake than in those with partial or no thallium uptake (Fig. 3).

2. Intracoronary technetium-99m pyrophosphate scintigraphy after thrombolysis

In about 20% of the patients, however, wall motion did not improve despite new thallium uptake. In these patients with false-positive thallium scintigrams pyrophosphate accumulated in the area of new thallium uptake (5, 8). An example is shown

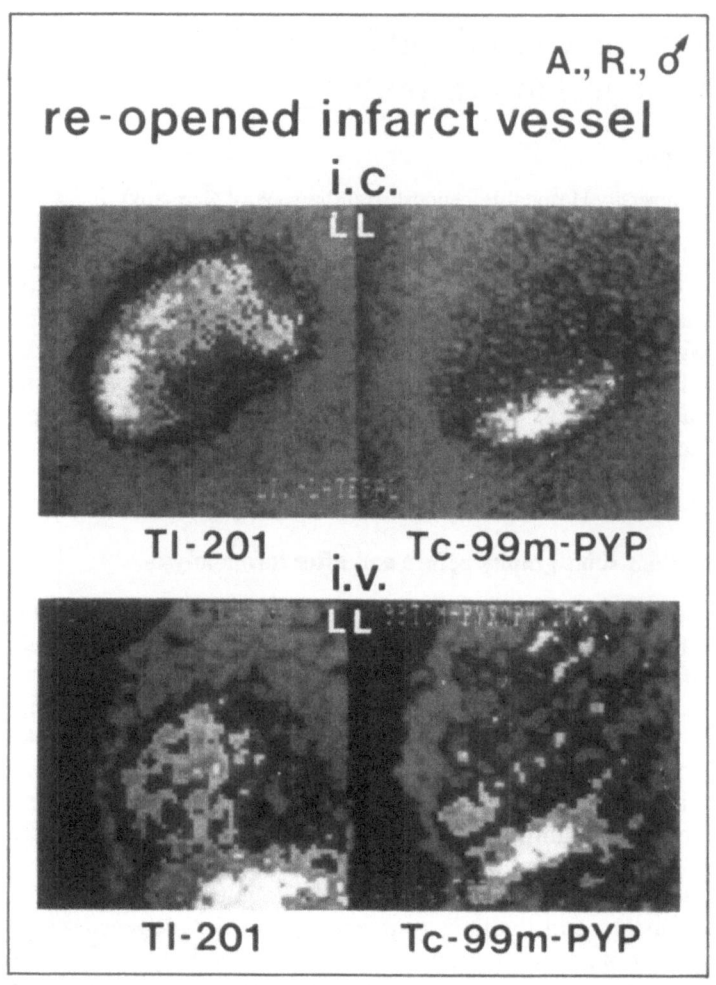

Fig. 1. Comparison of intracoronary (upper panel) with intravenous (lower panel) 201-thallium (Tl-201) and technetium (Tc-99m) pyrophosphate (PYP) scintigraphy. Note the high quality after intracoronary injection of the isotopes in this patient with an acute inferior infarction

in Fig. 4. In this patient thallium was taken up after thrombolysis in the interventricular septum. After intracoronary injection of pyrophosphate into the infarct vessel pyrophosphate accumulated in the area of new thallium uptake. To exclude the possibility that this thallium/pyrophosphate overlap was the result of superimposition from different layers of different depths we performed emission computed tomography in these patients, clearly revealing the close neighbourhood of viable and necrotic cells. The clinical significance of this finding is that wall motion will remain depressed in the area of overlap, whereas in patients with new thallium uptake but no thallium/pyrophosphate overlap wall motion will improve (8).

In the context of these studies, we firstly could demonstrate in patients that pyrophosphate accumulates immediately after re-opening of an infarct vessel in the ne-

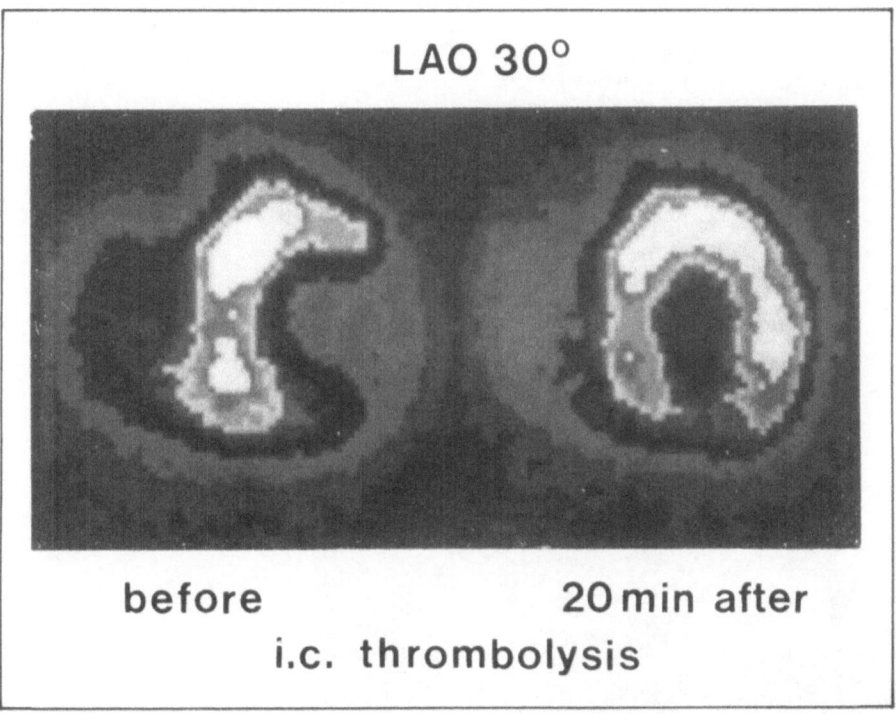

Fig. 2. Intracoronary Tl-201 scintigrams before and 20 minutes after thrombolysis in a patient with an antero-lateral infarction. There is complete new Tl-201 uptake in the defect area after reopening of the infarct artery and i.c. Tl-201 reinfarction

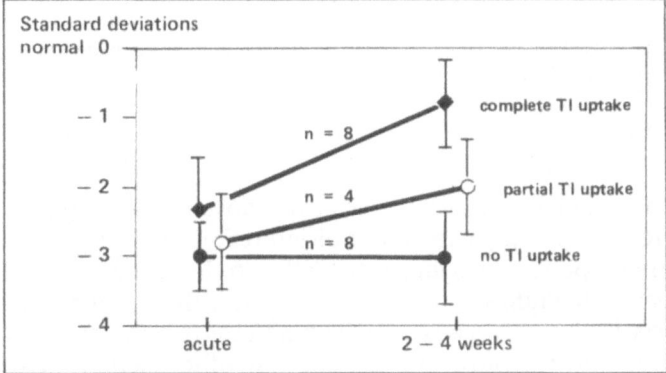

Fig. 3. Relationship between wall motion in the infarct area (acute and follow-up) and new Tl-201 uptake immediately after thrombolysis. Wall motion is expressed in standard deviations from normal: values of less than −2 SD indicate severe hypokinesis. New Tl-201 uptake immediately after thrombolysis is related to follow-up wall motion

135

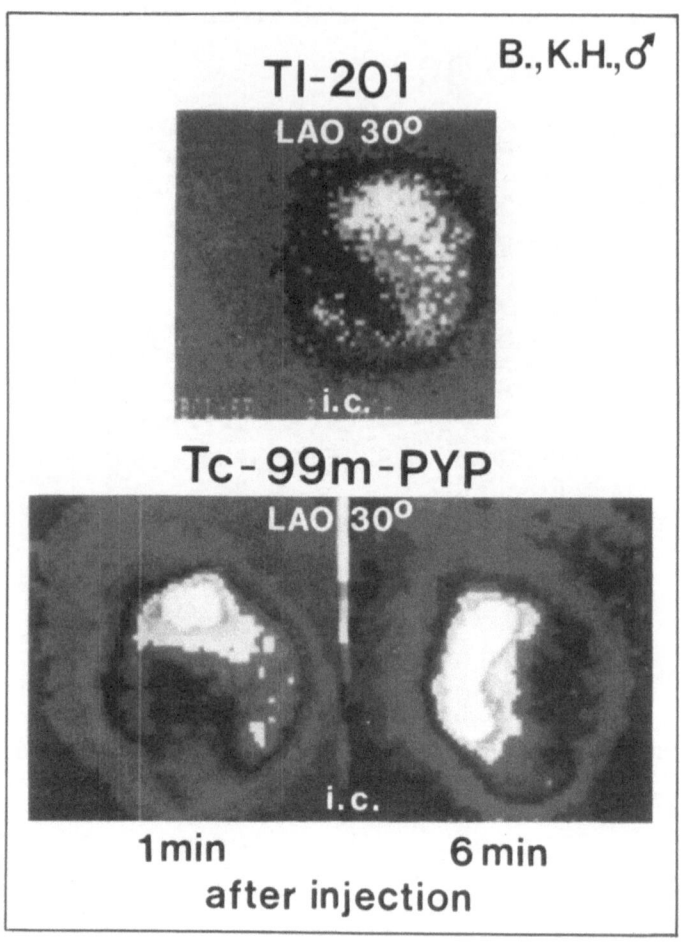

Fig. 4. This figure illustrates the acute pyrophosphate accumulation in the infarct area in the presence of a patent infarct artery. In this patient with a septal Tl-201 defect after thrombolysis, one minute after injection Tc-99m PYP is distributed according to perfusion to the non-ischemic area. Six minutes later, pyrophosphate is already washed out from these regions now accumulating in the acutely infarcted segment [with permission of the European Heart Journal (7)]

crotic tissue, whereas in conventionally treated patients pyrophosphate scintigraphy becomes positive only 12 to 24 hours after the onset of infarction (6). Early pyrophosphate accumulation after reperfusion is illustrated in Fig. 5. In the upper panel of this figure, an intracoronary thallium scintigram in a patient with an anterior infarct shows a residual defect in the interventricular septum immediately after successful thrombolysis. One minute after intracoronary injection of technetium pyrophosphate, this isotope was distributed similarly to thallium, reflecting perfusion at this time. Six minutes later, pyrophosphate has already been washed out from the viable myocardium. It now accumulates in the infarct area, the interventricular septum which is also the area of the residual thallium defect.

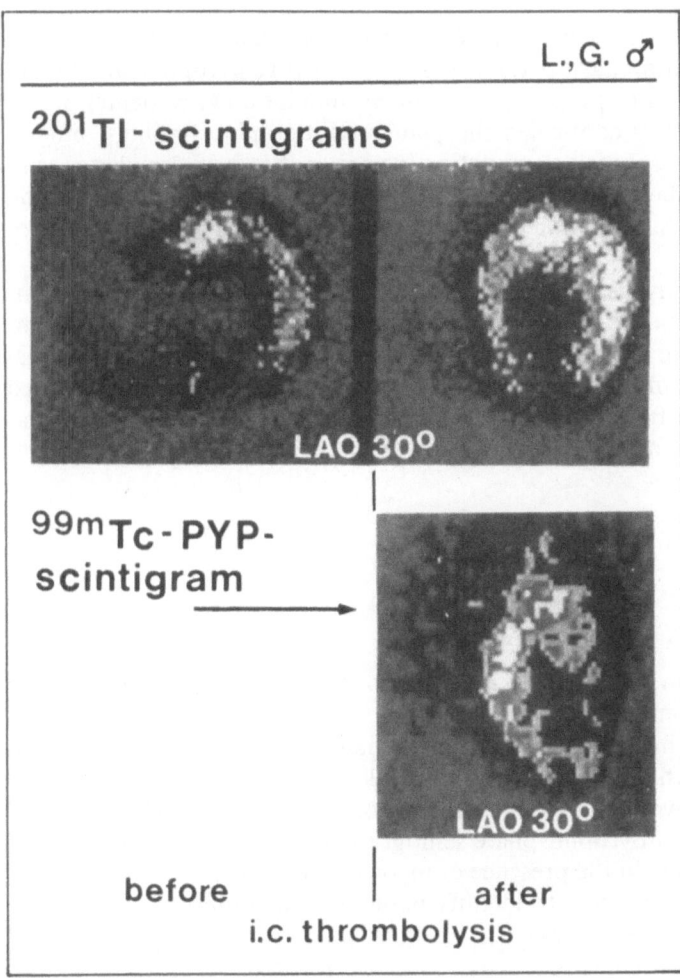

L., G. ♂

^{201}Tl- scintigrams

LAO 30°

^{99m}Tc - PYP-
scintigram →

LAO 30°

before | after
i.c. thrombolysis

Fig. 5. Overlap of Tl-201 uptake and Tc-99m pyrophosphate accumulation. After thrombolysis, new Tl-201 uptake is noted in the interventricular septum. Tc-99m pyrophosphate also accumulates in the interventricular septum reflecting the close neighbourhood of viable and necrotic cells [with permission of the Journal of the American College of Cardiology (5)]

3. Early intravenous technetium-99m pyrophosphate scintigraphy after thrombolysis

The early accumulation of pyrophosphate in the presence of a patent infarct artery suggests that reperfusion may be assessed non-invasively by early pyrophosphate scintigraphy. If so, this would be very important for intravenous thrombolysis, since other non-invasive methods such as the electrocardiogram and enzymatic methods have failed to reliably indicate reperfusion in the individual patient. We addressed this problem by giving 10 mCi technetium pyrophosphate intravenously to 14 patients within the first hours after intravenous thrombolysis. All patients underwent acute and follow-up coronary and left ventricular angiography (7). In the 4 patients

137

with an occluded infarct vessel early pyrophosphate scintigraphy was negative. In the presence of a patent infarct artery there was either massive pyrophosphate accumulation (5 patients), focal or no pyrophosphate accumulation (7 patients). Computed emission tomography confirmed the planar scintigraphic findings, but revealed faint focal pyrophosphate accumulation in some patients whose planar scintigrams were negative. These data suggest that early pyrophosphate accumulation may be used as a non-invasive method to indicate reperfusion in the presence of myocardial necrosis.

Can early PYP-scintigraphy also be used to estimate definite infarct size after thrombolysis? To address this question we compared left ventricular wall motion in the infarct area during the acute and follow-up state. In patients with massive pyrophosphate accumulation wall motion was markedly depressed and remained depressed at follow-up. In the reperfused patients with little focal pyrophosphate accumulation, however, wall motion at the infarct site was better initially with further improvement at follow-up.

4. Conclusions

These studies show:
1. Intracoronary thallium scintigraphy is useful to determine myocardial salvage immediately after thrombolysis.
2. The additional use of intracoronary pyrophosphate helps to identify patients in whom intracoronary thallium scintigraphy is false-positive. (Patients with thallium/pyrophosphate overlap in whom wall motion will remain depressed.)
3. Intravenous technetium/pyrophosphate scintigraphy may be useful to detect reperfusion non-invasively in the presence of myocardial necrosis.
4. I.v. PYP-scintigraphy may help to identify patients with compromised left ventricular function after thrombolysis.

References

1. Mathey DG et al (1981) Intracoronary streptokinase thrombolytic recanalization and subsequent surgical bypass of remaining atherosclerotic stenosis in acute myocardial infarction: complementary combined approach effecting reduced infarct size, preventing reinfarction, and improving left ventricular function. Am Heart J 102:1194
2. Mathey DG et al (1983) Use of streptokinase in coronary thrombosis. In: Hurst JW (ed) Clinical essays on the heart. McGraw-Hill, New York, pp 203–224
3. Merx W et al (1981) Evaluation of the effectiveness of intracoronary streptokinase infusion in acute myocardial infarction: postprocedure management and hospital course in 204 patients. Am Heart J 102:1181
4. Meyer J et al (1982) Percutaneous transluminal coronary angioplasty immediately after intracoronary streptolysis of transmural myocardial infarction. Circulation 66:905–913
5. Schofer J et al (1983) Use of dual scintigraphy with thallium-201 and technetium-99m pyrophosphate to predict improvement in left ventricular wall motion immediately after intracoronary thrombolysis in acute myocardial infarction. J Am Coll Cardiol 2:737
6. Schofer J et al (1984) Assessment of myocardial necrosis immediately after intracoronary thrombolysis by intracoronary injection of technetium-99m pyrophosphate. Eur Heart J 5:617

7. Schofer J et al (1985) Intravenöse Technetium-99m Pyrophosphat-Szintigraphie zum frühzeiti-
   gen Nachweis einer Reperfusion beim akuten Myokardinfarkt. Z Kardiol 74 (Suppl 5):65
8. Schofer J et al (1985) Thallium-201/technetium-99m pyrophosphate overlap in patients with
   acute myocardial infarction after thrombolysis predicts depressed wall motion despite thallium
   uptake. Am Heart J (in press)

Authors' address:

D. G. Mathey, M.D.
Department of Cardiology
University Hospital Eppendorf
Martinistr. 52
2000 Hamburg 20
West Germany

Echocardiography in myocardial infarction

R. Erbel, H. J. Rupprecht, B. Henkel, K. J. Henrichs, and J.Meyer

II. Medical Clinic, Johannes Gutenberg-University, Mainz (West Germany)

This paper discusses the usefulness of echocardiography in thrombolysis, its diagnostic value and drawbacks for therapy and the possibilities for follow-up studies. The diagnostic value is seen in the possibility of localizing and defining the extent of myocardial infarction, not only of the left but also of the right ventricle, and recognizing the complications of myocardial infarction as soon as possible 1, 2, 4.

In 14 out of 242 patients transferred to our university, where we started or wanted to start thrombolysis, we found ECGs with ST segment elevation suggestive of acute transmural myocardial infarction. However, two-dimensional echocardiography revealed that wall motion was normal. Later, pericardial effusion developed enabling the diagnosis of pericarditis (Fig. 1).

In acute anterior myocardial infarction the ECG allows the estimation of the extent of the infarction in many patients. Figure 2 shows in a typical echocardiographic image akinesia of the apical region with systolic thinning. The basal parts of the left ventricle preserved normal function.

In lateral and inferior myocardial infarction the ECG-based estimation of infarct size is limited. In Fig. 3 only slight changes of the ECG are present, but CK rose to 1782 U/l.

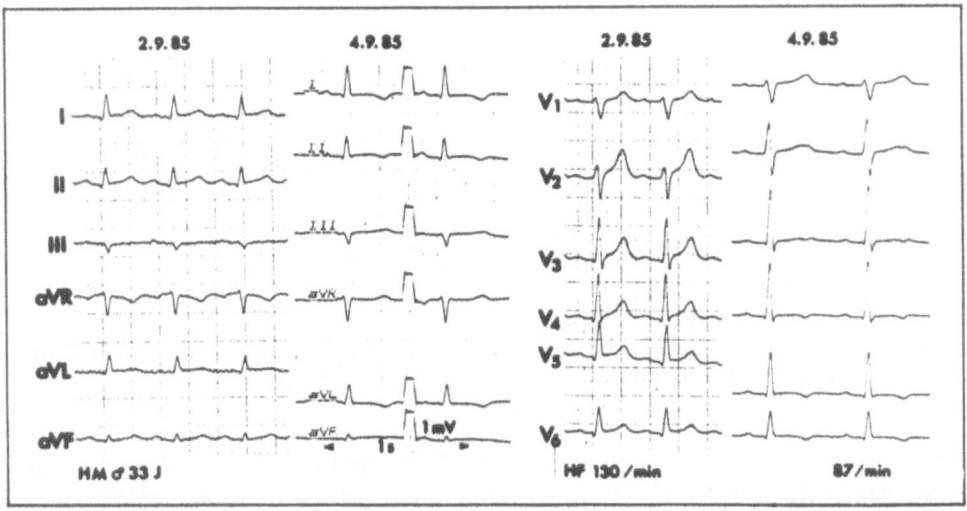

Fig. 1. ECG of a patient with acute pericarditis. In the acute stage the changes are suggestive of acute transmural anterior myocardial infarction. Follow-up demonstrated pericarditis with pericardial effusion

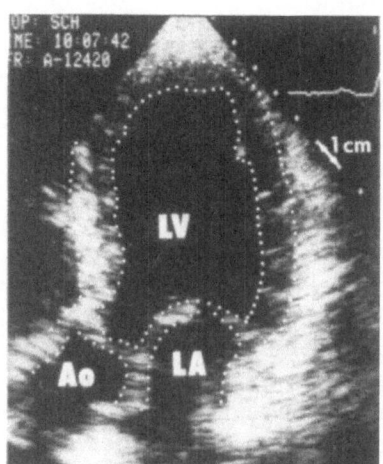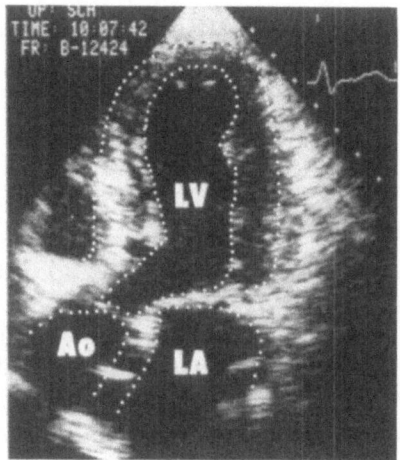

Fig. 2. End-diastolic and end-systolic apical RAO view demonstrating apical akinesia with good basal function of the left ventricle. Anterior wall and posterior wall demonstrate normal thickening. The apical region demonstrates wall thinning. LA/LV = left atrium/left ventricle, Ao = Aorta

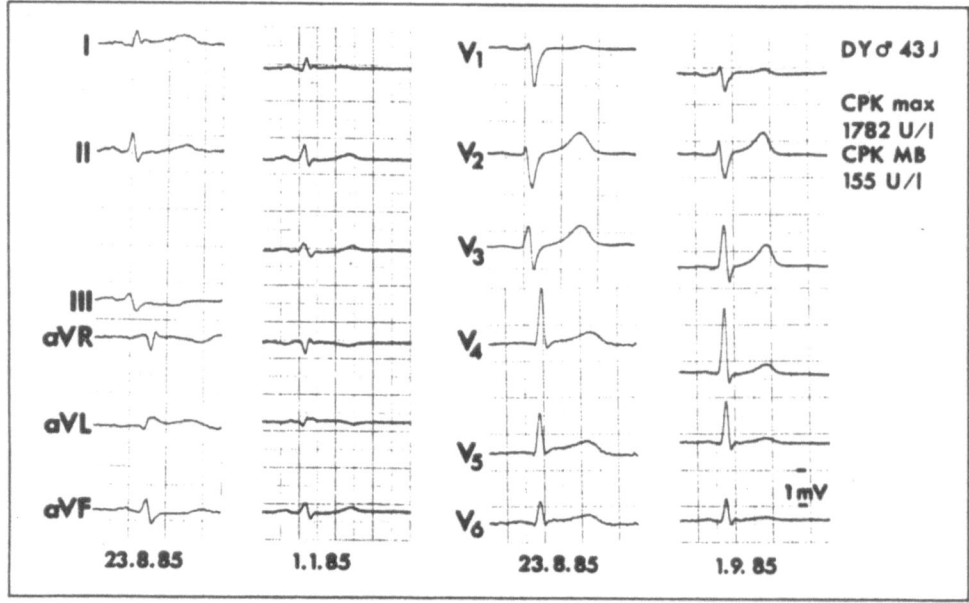

Fig. 3. ECG of a patient with extended lateral myocardial infarction. Whereas in the ECG only minor changes in I and AVL can be observed, CPK increases to 1782 μ/l

A particular problem exists with patients who have right ventricle involvement in inferior myocardial infarction. By two-dimensional echocardiography, performed at the coronary care unit or in the catheterization laboratory, we can recognize very quickly if the anterior wall of the right ventricle has a disturbed wall motion. Figures 4 and 5 show an apical four chamber view and a cross-sectional short axis

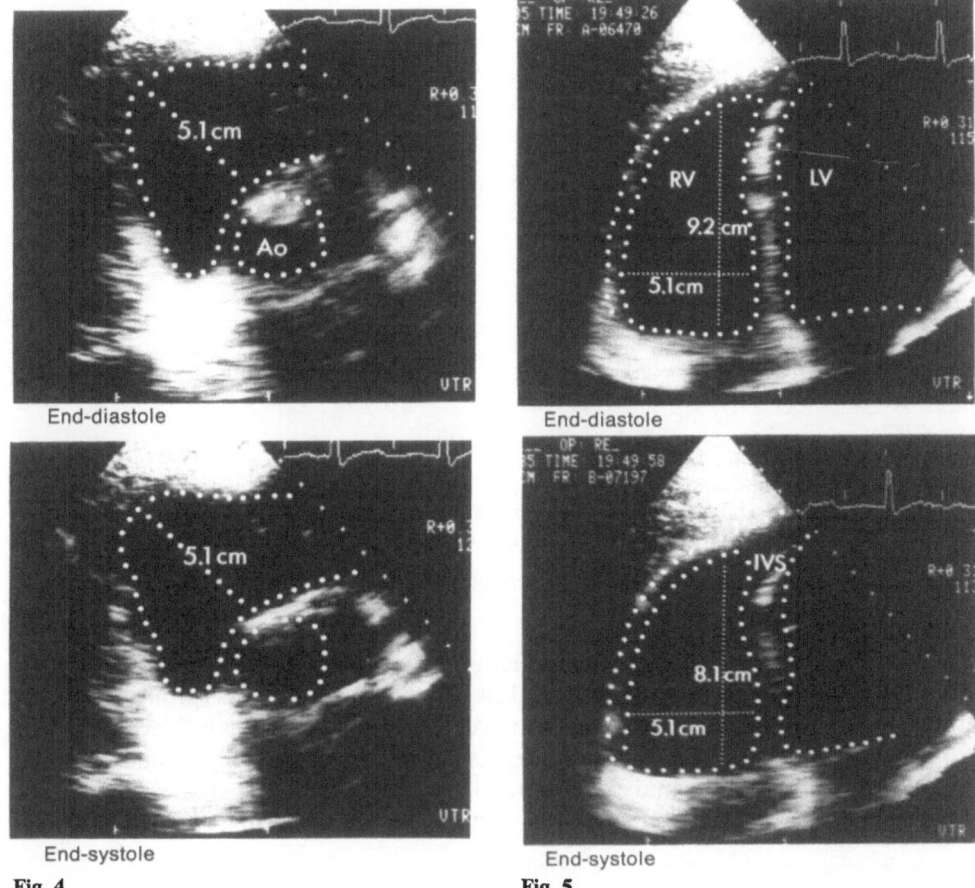

End-diastole   End-diastole

End-systole   End-systole

Fig. 4   **Fig. 5**

Fig. 4. End-diastolic and end-systolic left parasternal short axis view of the right ventricle. No shortening is present

Fig. 5. Apical four chamber view. In right ventricular infarction no shortening of the diameter, only shortening of the long axis from end-diastole to end-systole is present

view. Using this method we have found it possible to show disturbed wall motion in 30 of 71 patients with inferior myocardial infarction. It can be seen from Fig. 5 that there is no shortening of the diameter of the right ventricle. Only shortening of the long axis occurred because the apical part of the right ventricle is supplied by the left anterior descending coronary artery and the anterior wall is supplied by the right occluded coronary artery. In terms of hemodynamics (Fig. 6a, b), patients with right ventricular involvement had lower systolic blood pressure, heart rate and cardiac index and higher right atrial blood pressure than patients with inferior myocardial infarction without involvement of the right ventricle. After four weeks and thrombolysis therapy right ventricular function had significantly improved. Thus, two-dimensional echocardiography correctly identified a group of patients with involvement of the right ventricle which was confirmed by hemodynamic studies (5).

143

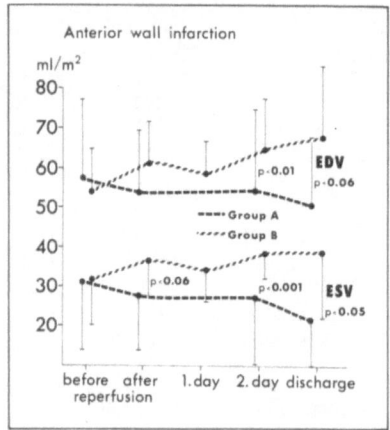

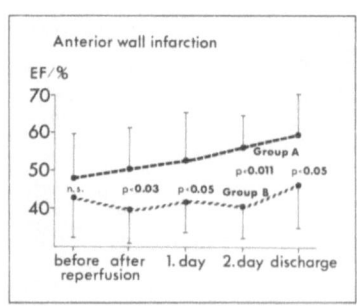

Fig. 6 a   **Fig. 6 b**

Fig. 6 a. Changes of end-diastolic and end-systolic volume (EDV/ESV) in patients with anterior myocardial infarction with short infarct time (group A 3 h 30 min) and long infarct time (group B more than 3 h 3 min) before, after reperfusion at the first and second day and before discharge (2)

Fig. 6 b. Changes of the left ventricular ejection fraction for the groups demonstrated in Fig. 6a (2)

The effect of thrombolysis therapy on left ventricular function in 54 patients with anterior wall infarction is demonstrated in Fig. 6 a, b. In patients (group B) with a long infarct time, i.e. an infarct time up to reperfusion of more than three and a half hours, immediately after reperfusion there is a trend towards increased end-diastolic and end-systolic volumes, and ejection fraction decreased (6). In patients with a short infarct time, ejection fraction improved significantly, and end-diastolic and end-sys-

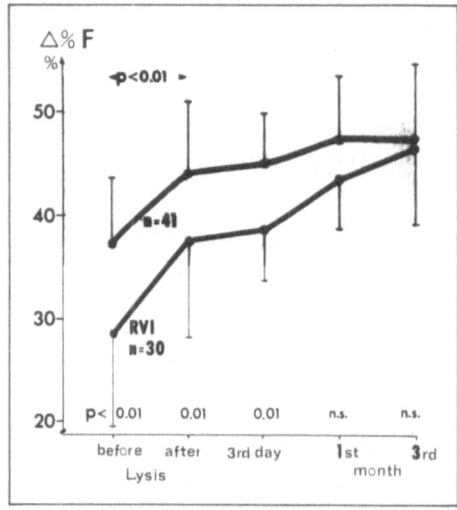

Fig. 7. Changes of shortening fraction of the right ventricular area (%F) in patients with (n = 30) and without (n = 41) involvement of the right ventricle in inferior myocardial infarction during follow-up to three months (6)

144

tolic volumes decreased yielding improved ventricular function. In patients with involvement of the right ventricle, immediately after thrombolysis recovery of ventricular function occurred. Three months later, patients with and without involvement of the right ventricle were not significantly different (Fig. 7).

Angiographic and two-dimensional echocardiographic data in the acute stage and before discharge were compared. In a group with anterior myocardial infarction in whom both thrombolysis and PTCA were carried out, despite a difference in absolute values, changes of volumes and ejection fraction were similar. In patients with inferior myocardial infarction and thrombolysis therapy with PTCA, despite differences in absolute values, the direction of changes of volumes and particularly ejection fraction was comparable.

Regional wall motion evaluated by both methods was compared in patients with thrombolysis therapy and PTCA. The results in anterior myocardial infarction and in the group without PTCA demonstrated an insignificant increase of wall motion from the acute to the chronic stage. The differences between the acute and the control study before discharge were much greater in the group with thrombolysis and PTCA. These changes were significant in 7 segments of the anterior wall. Not only for the global function but also for regional wall motion in group comparisons, two-dimensional echocardiography is capable of describing changes similar to those observed by cineventriculography (3).

Summary

For two-dimensional echocardiography qualitative analysis can be performed in 90% of patients and a quantitative analysis of the left ventricle in 75%. Two-dimensional echocardiography has the advantage that it can be performed prior to the recanalization procedure without delay, while the catheterization procedure is prepared. This process can reveal data relevant to diagnosis and with consequences for therapy. Of course a disadvantage is the low resolution and a high interobserver variability but newer techniques, such as contrast echocardiography and transducer with annular array offer the prospect of better resolution in the future. On the other hand, cineventriculography has the disadvantage that contrast medium has negative inotropic effects and volume loading. Particularly follow-up studies are limited. In the future more information will be available from echocardiography, including flow measurements by Doppler and coronary perfusion examinations by contrast echocardiography. In addition, new information from tissue type texture analysis can be expected.

References

1. Charuzi Y, Beeder C, Marshall L, Sasaki H, Pack N, Geft J, Ganz W (1984) Improvement of regional and global left ventricular function after intracoronary thrombolysis: Assessment with two-dimensional echocardiography. Am J Cardiol 53:662–665
2. Erbel R (1985) Funktionsdiagnostik des linken Ventrikels. In: Grube E (ed) Zweidimensionale Echokardiographie. Thieme Verlag, Stuttgart, pp 345–368

3. Erbel R, Pop T, Meinertz T, Clas W, Henkel B, Schreiner G, Steuernagel C, Meyer J (1984) Analysis of left ventricular function before and immediately after recanalization in acute myocardial infarction. Eur Heart J 5 (Suppl I):220
4. Erbel R, Brennecke R, Clas W, Henkel B, Henrichs KJ, Steuernagel C, Meyer J (1985) Infarktbestimmung mittels Echokardiographie. In: Kleinsorge H, Schölmerich P (eds) Apparative versus medikamentöse Therapie in der Kardiologie. Gustav Fischer Verlag, Stuttgart New York, pp 141–149
5. Henrichs KJ, Erbel R, Steuernagel C, Meyer J (1985) Improvement of myocardial perfusion by thrombolysis evaluation of left ventricular function by two-dimensional echocardiography. In: Meyer J, Erbel R, Rupprecht HJ (eds) Improvement of myocardial perfusion. Martinus Nijhoff Publishers, Dordrecht, pp 104–111
6. Rupprecht HJ, Erbel R, Schöer KH, Schreiner GH, Henrichs KL, Meyer J (1985) Right ventricular infarction: Echocardiographic, hemodynamic feature. In: Meyer J, Erbel R, Rupprecht HJ (eds) Improvement of myocardial perfusion. Martinus Nijhoff Publishers, Dordrecht, pp 112–124

Author's address:
Prof. Dr. med. R. Erbel
II. Medizinische Klinik und Poliklinik
Klinikum der Johannes-Gutenberg-Universität
Langenbeckstraße 1
6500 Mainz
West Germany

Discussion

HUGENHOLTZ:

I do not disagree on the potential promise of echocardiography and its advantage over angiography and other techniques, but we need techniques than can be tried under battlefield conditions. Although we have plenty of echo apparatus in our unit, we do not seem to be able to get the information at the bedside when the clinician needs it. Have you been able in your unit to set up a pragmatic arrangement so that the interobserver variation over twenty-four hours is sufficiently evened out that the data can be trusted when they are required?

ERBEL:

When we began two years ago we had two teams doing thrombolysis therapy, and in each team carrying out heart catheterization we included one person who was capable of doing 2-D studies by himself, so that we had no technician or additional person for doing these studies. We therefore had a special program and we are well used to doing these volume studies, but are of course limited by the number of patients we have to exclude: up to a quarter of the patients cannot be studied.

Question:

Are experienced personnel like physicians required, or can technicans do this work?

ERBEL:

Physicians are necessary.

Question:

So we need physicians on service for twenty-four hours a day to achieve the results that you show us.

ERBEL:

Yes.

Remark:

I must say that echocardiography is the one technique which could allow the severity of the infarct to be gauged straight away, so it has that potential advantage over some of the other techniques.

How to estimate reocclusion risk?

R. Uebis

Department of Internal Medicine I, RWTH Aachen (West Germany)

Introduction

There are four main factors which may influence the incidence of reocclusion after previously successful thrombolysis in acute myocardial infarction:
On one hand, the "quality of reperfusion," that is the characteristics of blood flow into the ischemic myocardium and the time interval between onset of chest pain and successful reperfusion; both factors are in some way related to the anatomy of the lesion at the previous site of occlusion and the degree of residual stenosis (1, 2, 8, 12, 15, 16), that is the underlying coronary heart disease. On the other hand, the coagulatory system including variations in blood viscosity and other factors like vasospasm must be mentioned. To some extent, most of those components can be affected by drugs – consider calcium channel blockers for vasospasm – or other measures like for instance PTCA (4, 13, 14) or bypass surgery (11) to improve quality of reperfusion.
The literature suggests an incidence of reocclusion from about 10 to 30% (3, 6, 7, 9). The purpose of this study was not to give a review of data already published, but rather to analyse our own experience with nearly 600 patients, and to demonstrate some facilities which can be used to approach an estimation of reocclusion risk.

Patients and methods

So far, from a total of 543 patients treated with intracoronary thrombolysis because of acute myocardial infarction, the late clinical follow-up of 375 cases is available. The initial thrombolysis in the entire group was performed up to July 1984, the start of the 1st European rt-PA trial; methods have been extensively described elsewhere (5, 10).
Three days after the acute event – before the removal of the introducer sheet – a first control angiogram was obtained, and a second was obtained 6 months up to 2 years later (277/543 cases). Each angiogram was qualitatively analysed with regard to the patency of the infarct related vessel.
In addition, in a subgroup of 140 patients, the acute and first follow-up angiogram was assessed quantitatively using a Vanguard projector, contour finding by hand, and determination of diameter and cross sectional narrowing as well as concentricity, eccentricity and length of the lesion (Table 1). For this purpose, at least two radiological projections, usually perpendicular to each other, were analysed by an experienced assessor. Within the observation period, no PTCA or bypass operation was performed in this subgroup. "Reocclusion" in this context means nonfatal occlusion with or without clinical signs of reinfarction (i.e. recurrent ECG changes, en-

Table 1.

	Study group	Entire group
n	140	543
Age/years	56.2 ± 9	56.0 ± 10
♂/♀	124/16	478/65
Infarct related vessel/%		
LAD	42	46
RCx	15	13
RCA	39	38
other	4	3

zyme-release or angina pectoris). Patients who died within the control period were excluded, although death might have been due to reocclusion and fatal reinfarction. Thus, the true figure of the reocclusion rate will in fact be higher.

As a pilot trial in a small subgroup of patients, ST-segment changes were monitored continuously after successful thrombolysis by means of 6–8 precordial electrodes. Data processing including the measurement of ST-deviation 60 ms after the J point was performed using a fully computerized setting, derived from a multi-electrode precordial mapping system.

Medical therapy following successful thrombolysis routinely consisted of 24–30,000 IU of heparin/24 h within the first 3–5 days and cumarine or acetylic salicylic acid (500 mg/24 h) afterwards, nitrates and calcium channel blockers orally. β-blocking agents were given on indication only.

Results

1. Incidence of reocclusion and reinfarction

Within the first 3 days after successful thrombolysis, 8.5% of patients (24/277) suffered from reocclusion, documented in the first follow-up angiogram (Fig. 1); another 13.2% of patients (37/277) had reocclusion during the late follow-up period. Thus, a total amount of 21.7% of previously successfully reperfused infarct related vessels were assessed as non-patent.

Not every angiographically documented reocclusion resulted in reinfarction; there was a close relation to the initial time of ischemia (Fig. 2). Almost every patient with an initial duration of ischemia of less than 2 h suffered from symptomatic reinfarction, if reocclusion occurred; however, none of those patients in whom occlusion time exceeded 6 h had clear symptoms of reinfarction.

2. Residual stenosis after successful thrombolysis

In the subgroup of cases in which quantitative analysis of the residual lesion was performed (n = 140), the first angiogram revealed an average cross-section stenosis of

150

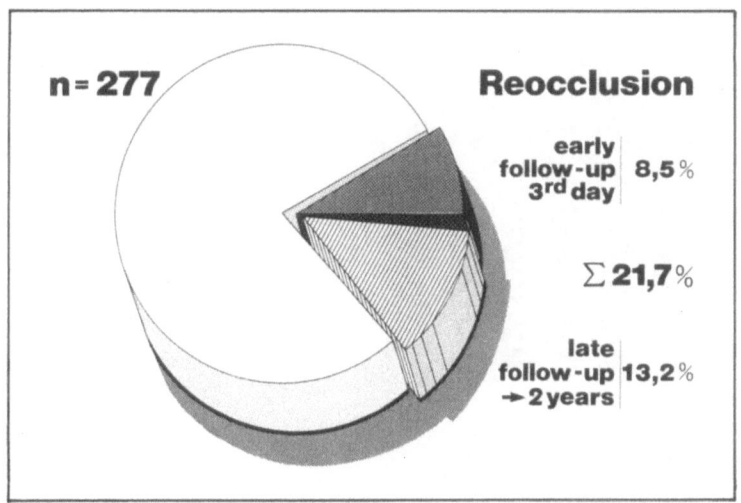

Fig. 1. Incidence of reocclusion following previously successful thrombolysis

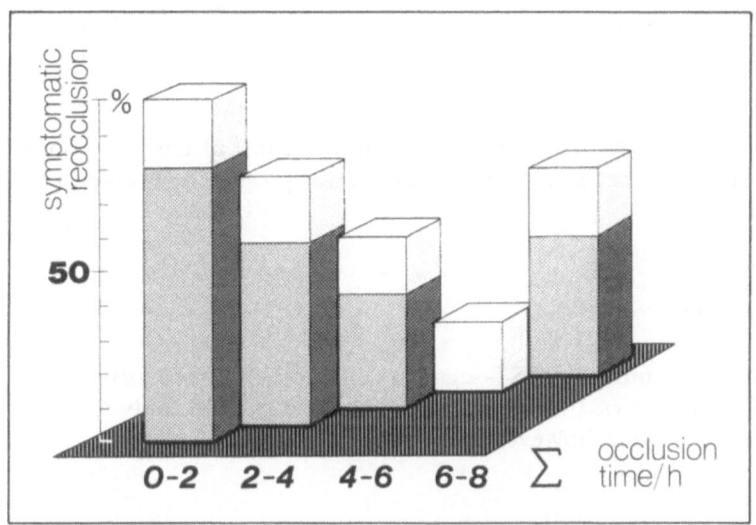

Fig. 2. Incidence of symptomatic vs. asymptomatic reocclusion.
Angiographically documented reocclusion *and* signs of reinfarction (i.e. new onset of angina pectoris, ST-segment elevation, or second rise in CK)
Angiographically documented reocclusion without signs of reinfarction.
Occlusion time: interval between onset of chest pain and successful reperfusion

$90.4 \pm 5.9\%$, which decreased to the control angiogram to $86.3 \pm 11.0\%$ ($p < 0.05$). However, in only 16% of patients did this decrease exceed 10% of cross-sectional area. Subgroup analysis is shown in Fig. 3; no statistically significant difference could be found comparing initially complete vs. incomplete thrombotic obstructions, concentric vs. eccentric stenoses, or short vs. long lesions. Only a multivariate analysis of the anatomy revealed a statistically different behaviour: eccentric lesions

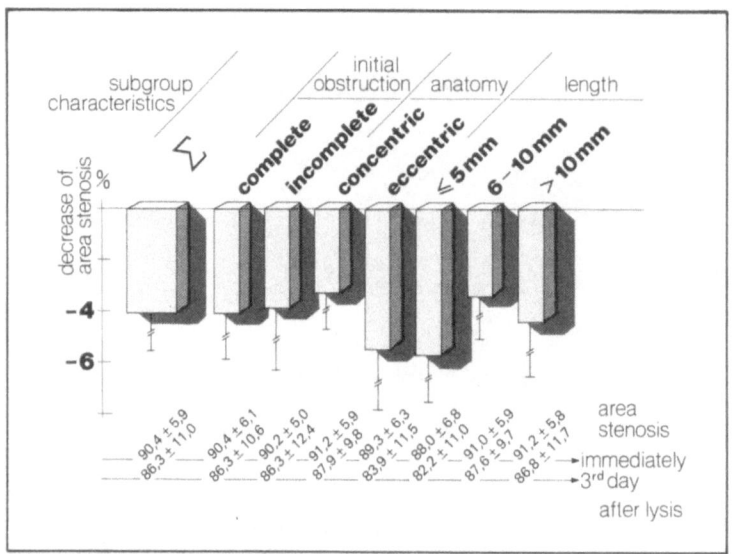

Fig. 3. Decrease of cross-sectional narrowing of the infarct related vessel after successful thrombolysis; subgroup analysis according to degree of initial obstruction, anatomy and length of the lesion

shorter than 5 mm decreased significantly more than in the rest of the study population (Fig. 4); however, this special anatomical setting was present in only 8 patients (5.8%) of the entire group.

3. ST-segment monitoring

By means of continuous monitoring of ST-segment deviation after successful thrombolysis, a plot of ST-changes vs. time course is possible. At present, only few individual case reports are available; however, recurrent ischemic episodes can be clearly recognized (Fig. 5).

Discussion

Despite "aggressive" anticoagulation, reocclusion and reinfarction still represent a major problem after previously successful thrombolysis. Methods to assess reocclusion risk in the individual patient at a very early stage after acute myocardial infarction are urgently needed. Clinical circumstances, the instantaneous ECG, ultrasound and scintigraphic techniques are not providing useful data concerning this problem. Continuous monitoring of the ST-segment may be useful for early detection of recurrent ischemia, but possibly too late to prevent reocclusion. In addition, more experience with larger numbers of patients is needed. Therefore, the only method to provide at least a few data is a quantitative analysis of a coronary angiogram, ob-

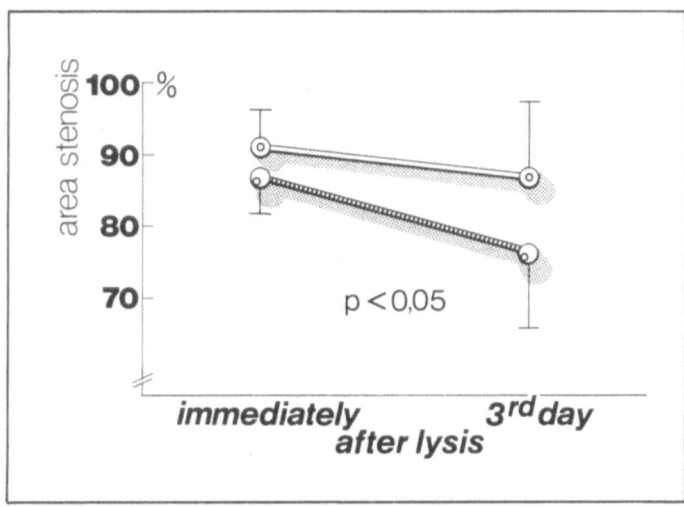

Fig. 4. Cross-sectional narrowing after thrombolysis:
⊚────⊚ concentric stenoses > 10 mm of length
⊚┄┄┄┄⊚ eccentric stenoses ≦ 5 mm of length

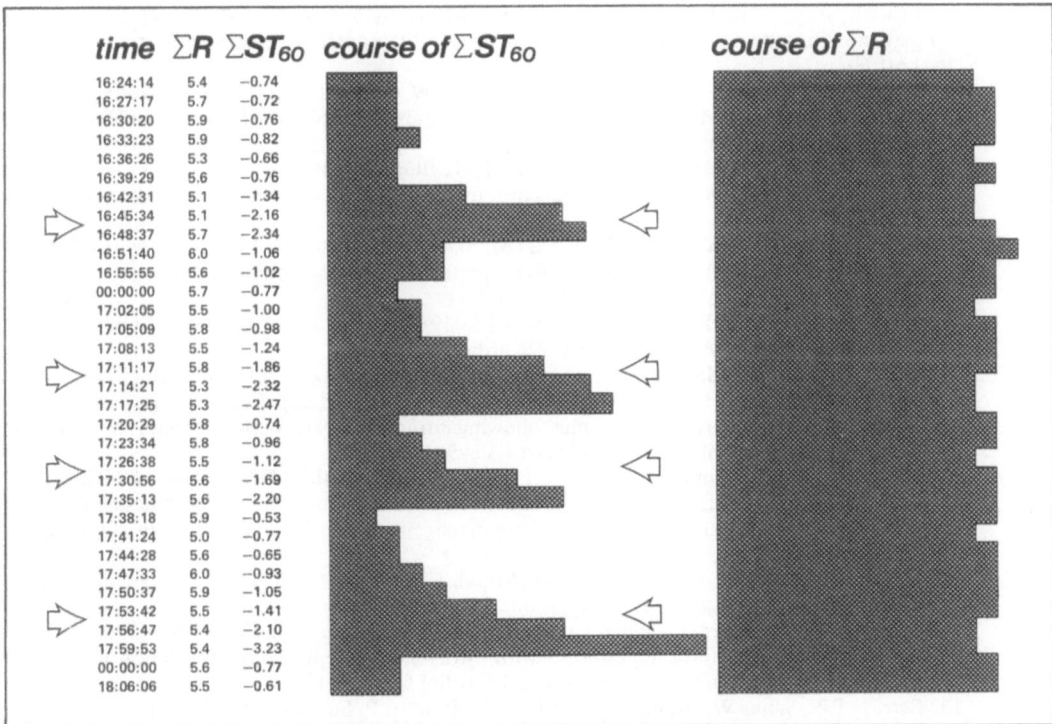

Fig. 5. Case report of continuous ST segment monitoring after successful thrombolysis
▷ Recurrent episodes of angina, associated with ST segment elevation (measured 60 ms after the j-point), but not with further decrase in R-wave amplitudes (course of R)

tained at a very early stage of acute myocardial infarction. The – rather small – subgroup of patients with initially incomplete thrombotic obstruction seems to be at lower reocclusion risk. Furthermore, eccentric and very short lesions show a significantly higher extent of decrease within the first 3 days after thrombolysis compared with others. However, only a small subgroup of patients is presenting with this very special anatomic situation.

The consequence is that scientific investigation of the near future will have to focus on two problems in this field: the development of safe criteria to predict reocclusion risks in the individual patients, and – at the same time – the testing of the efficacy of measures which could be capable of preventing reocclusion completely, such as PTCA, bypass surgery, or medical alternatives.

References

1. Brown BG, Bolson EL, Dodge HT (1984) Dynamic mechanism in human coronary stenosis. Circulation 70/6:917–922
2. Cribier A, Saoudi N, Berland J, Letac B (1985) Régression de la sténose coronaire résiduelle après récanalisation par fibrinolyse dans l'infarctus du myocarde. Arch Mal Coeur 3:353–360
3. Dörr R, Essen R v, Uebis R, Schmidt WG, Lambertz H, Effert S (1986) Symptomatic and asymptomatic coronary reocclusion after successful reperfusion in relation to the initial time of transmural myocardial ischemia. JACC 7/2:22 A
4. Erbel R, Pop T, Henrichs KJ, Rupprecht HJ, Meyer J (1985) Immediate angioplasty after reperfusion in acute myocardial infarction – a prospective controlled randomised trial. Eur Heart J 6/1:60
5. Essen R v, Uebis R, Schmidt WG, Dörr R, Merx W, Meyer J, Effert S, Schweizer P, Erbel R, Bardos P, Minale C, Messmer BJ (1985) Intrakoronare Streptokinase beim akuten Herzinfarkt. Dtsch med Wschr 110:570–575
6. Gold HK, Leinbach RC, Palacios IF, Yasuda T, Block PC, Buckley MJ, Akins CW, Daggett WM, Austen WG (1983) Coronary reocclusion after selective administration of SK. Circulation 68/2:150–154
7. Harrison DG, Ferguson DSW, Collins STM, Skorton DJ, Ericksen EE, Kioschos JM, Marcus ML, White CW (1984) Rethrombosis after reperfusion with streptokinase: importance of geometry of residual lesions. Circulation 69/5:991–999
8. Karsch KR, Niemczyk P, Voelker W, Seipel L (1984) Dynamik der kritischen Stenose bei Patienten mit instabiler Angina pectoris. Z Kardiol 73:552–559
9. Lee C, Low RI, Takeda P, Joe P, DeMaria AN, Amsterdam EZ, Lui H, Dietrich P, Lee K, Mason DT (1982) Importance of follow-up medical and surgical approaches to prevent reinfarction, reocclusion, and recurrent angina following intracoronary thrombolysis with streptokinase in acute myocardial infarction. Am Heart J 104:921–924
10. Merx W, Dörr R, Rentrop P, Blanke H, Karsch KR, Mathey DG, Kremer P, Rutsch W, Schmutzler H (1981) Evaluation of the effectiveness of intracoronary streptokinase infusion in acute myocardial infarction: Postprocedure management and hospital course in 204 patients. Am Heart J 102:1181–1187
11. Messmer BJ, Merx W, Meyer J, Bardos P, Minale C, Effert S (1983) New developments in medical-surgical treatment of AMI. Ann Thorac Surg 35:70–78
12. Schröder R, Vöhringer H, Linderer T, Biamino G, Brüggemann T, Leitner ER v (1985) Follow-up after coronary arterial reperfusion with intravenous streptokinase in relation to residual myocardial infarct artery narrowings. Am J Cardiol 55:313–317
13. Serruys PW, Wijns W, Brand M vd, Ribeiro V, Fioretti P, Simoons ML, Kooijman CJ, Reiber JW, Hugenholtz PG (1983) Is transluminal coronary angioplasty mandatory after successful thrombolysis? Quantitative coronary angiographic study. Br Heart J 50:257–265
14. Swan HJC (1982) Thrombolysis in AMI: Treatment of the underlying CAD. Circulation 66:914–916

15. Uebis R, Essen R v, Schmidt WG, Franke A, Effert S (1985) Reststenose nach erfolgreicher selektiver Lyse kompletter thrombotischer Koronararterienverschlüsse beim akuten Myokardinfarkt. Z Kardiol 74:519–24
16. Voelker W, Karsch KR, Konz KH, Jacksch R, Schick KD, Risler T, Haasis R, Ickrath O, Hartmann S, Blanke H, Rentrop P, Seipel L (1984) Die spontane Regression der Reststenose des Infarktgefäßes nach erfolgreicher perkutaner transluminaler Koronarrekanalisation (PTCR). Z Kardiol 73:634–40

Author's address:
R. Uebis, M.D.
Klinikum der RWTH
Abteilung Innere Medizin I
Pauwelsstraße
5100 Aachen
West Germany

155

Indications for early PTCA after thrombolysis

J. Meyer, R. Erbel, T. Pop, and H. J. Rupprecht

Klinikum der Johannes Gutenberg-Universität Mainz (West Germany)

There are several ways to reopen an acutely occluded coronary artery. Thrombolysis can be achieved with various methods (1, 5, 7, 10). After thrombolysis we find that the residual thrombus can sometimes be seen, but in most cases, a more or less high grade coronary stenosis remains (2). It is also a question of whether it is always optimal to reopen the vessel, because if the vessel remains occluded, another occlusion cannot occur. With this situation one faces the possibility that the patient will suffer another infarction, and that the vessel will occlude again (4).

In about 75–80% of all successful thrombolysis cases, the coronary vessel remains highly stenosed. If PTCA is carried out for the same stenosis, then we may improve the blood flow to this previously ischemic area, and may further reduce the infarct size. We may also prevent a reocclusion, or may reduce the anginal symptoms after infarction because of the high grade stenosis in the ischemic areas (3, 6). Probably we may improve early and late prognosis and if the PTCA is done in the same session, as has been our practice since 1980, the patient is saved considerable inconvenience. We also further save time and money.

In Table 1 the results of our preliminary studies in Mainz concerning hospital mortality are detailed. We will only focus attention on these numbers. Following thrombolysis without PTCA reinfarctions occurred on days 2, 3, 4, 7, 8 and 17. Two cardiac ruptures occurred on day 2. One patient had asystole on the first day. There was one cardiac death and one cardiac shock. After PTCA, there were two reinfarctions on day 2, one cardiac rupture and three cases of cardiogenic shock on day 1. This means you cannot predict on what day a reinfarction will occur. Therefore, there is no

Table 1. Hospital mortality after thrombolysis. Group I: thrombolysis without PTCA; group II: thrombolysis with immediate PTCA

Group I 79 patients		Group II 83 patients	
Clinical picture	Day	Clinical picture	Day
6 reinfarctions	2, 3, 4, 7, 8, 17	2 reinfarctions	2
2 cardiac ruptures	2, 2	1 cardiac rupture	14
1 asystole	1	3 cardiogenic shock	1, 1, 1
1 sudden death	13		
1 cardiogenic shock	1		
1 pneumonia	22	3 shock lung	7, 9, 13
1 cerebral bleeding	7	1 cerebral bleeding	1
11/79 pts cardiac reasons (14%)		6/83 pts cardiac reasons (7%)	
2/79 pts non cardiac reasons (3%)		4/83 pts non cardiac reasons (5%)	

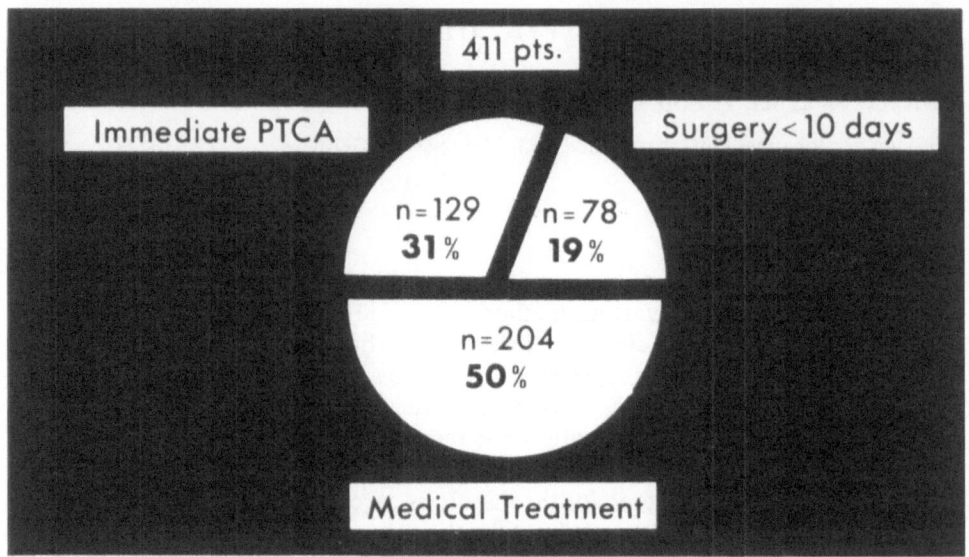

Fig. 1. Subsequent treatment after lysis in patients with acute myocardial infarction and successful thrombolysis (Aachen, West Germany). [From (3)]

possibility of predicting at what time PTCA should be done, or, in multi-vessel disease, when a bypass operation should be done. Thus, although we try to improve the coagulation system with cumadine and other methods, some patients have reinfarction quite early.

For this reason we carry out PTCA immediately (6). Figure 1 is a pie chart of the study reported by von Essen, presenting our results gathered in Aachen up to 1985 (3). From a total of 411 patients with successful lysis 78 (19%) were found to be suitable for bypass surgery and 129 (31%) were candidates for immediate PTCA, which was carried out straight away and in one session. Nowadays, I think we would

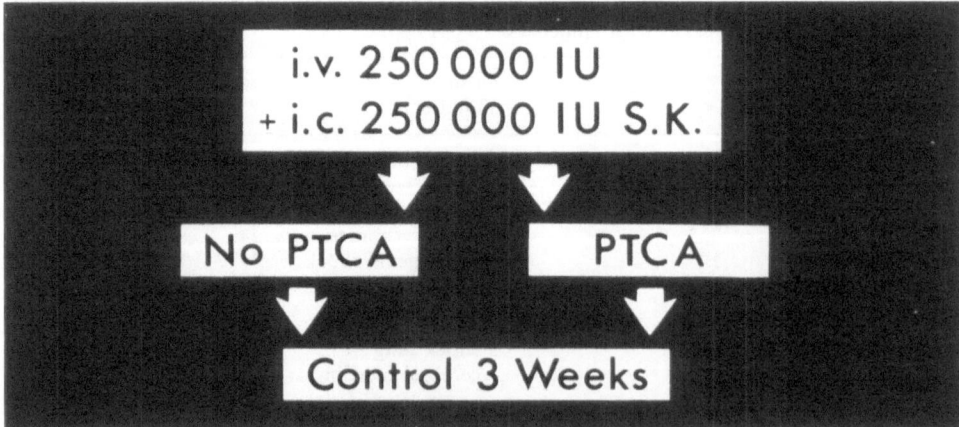

Fig. 2. Randomized study of thrombolysis with and without PTCA (Mainz, West Germany)

also treat several of the patients judged suitable for medical treatment by PTCA, since the balloons have improved so much. We would now include more patients with more irregular stenosis than we did in 1980.

Having shown that PTCA could be carried out in one third of patients we made a randomized study to prove that it was worthwhile (Fig. 2). All patients received intravenous and intracoronary streptokinase, so that there was no placebo group. Each patient received streptokinase, but one group had PTCA while the other did not. 79 patients (Group I) had no PTCA and 83 (Group II) were treated with PTCA. All patients were randomized, with no difference in ages and sex distribution and there was no upper age limit. There was no difference in the infarct size and its location.

In Group II (Fig. 3) we attempted to treat all patients with PTCA (streptokinase plus the guide wire technique), resulting in a recanalization rate of 86%. In only 65% was the attempted PTCA successful. This rate is much lower than in the normal PTCA but these were severely diseased vessels and we had the intention to treat. In 32% the treatment was unsuccessful, and in two patients another vessel occlusion was caused by the manipulation of the balloon. So in 3% of the cases there was a mechanical reocclusion caused by the balloon. This rate is rather low, and is the same as in our studies with stable and unstable angina.

On analysis of the results after three weeks, at the end of the hospital phase, we found an initial reperfusion rate in the group without PTCA of 90% and in the group with PTCA of 86% (Table 2). The success rate of PTCA was 65%. During the hospital phase there was a reocclusion rate of 18% in the group without PTCA compared to 12% in the group with PTCA. Reinfarction rate was 11% compared to 5%; lethal reinfarctions were 8% compared to 2%; and cardiac deaths were 14% compared to 7%. These figures are too low to be significant but the tendency seems to be that im-

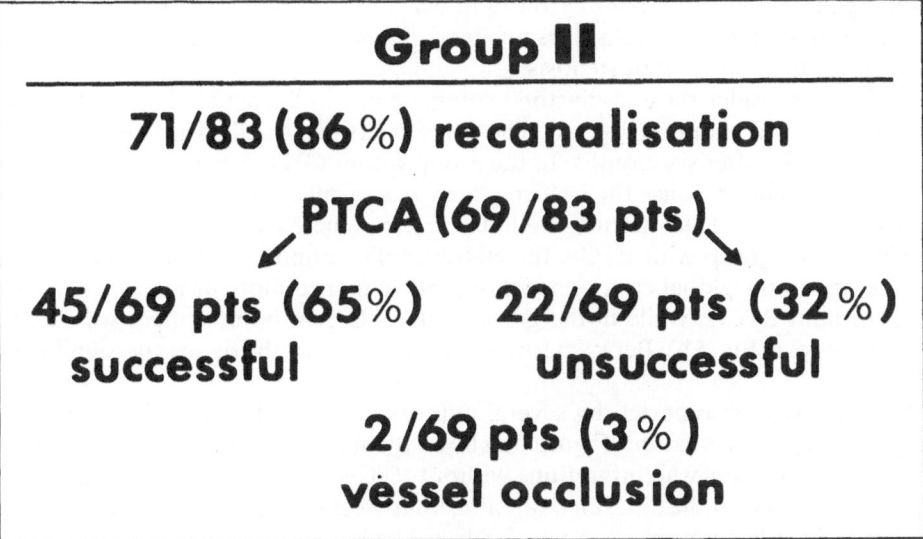

Fig. 3. Results of group II (thrombolysis with PTCA)

Table 2. Clinical results during the hospital phase after thrombolysis without and with PTCA

	Lysis without PTCA n = 79	Lysis with PTCA n = 83
Reperfusion rate	90%	86%
PTCA success	–	65%
Reocclusions	18%	12%
Reinfarctions	11%	5%
Reinfarctions (lethal)	8%	2%
Cardiac death	14%	7%

mediate PTCA, despite the risk of reocclusion, appears to be beneficial with respect to reocclusion rate, reinfarction, and also cardiac death.

Turning to the degree of the stenosis, Fig. 4a and b show the stenosis diameter in per cent in the group with successful dilatation (Fig. 4a) and the group without dilatation (Fig. 4b). Immediately after lysis and before dilatation, the rate was 81%. In some cases dilatation reduced the diameter dramatically to less than 20%. After four weeks there is some restenosis, but the average is the same as after PTCA, 32% vs. 29%. In the group without PTCA, where we did nothing apart from administering heparin and cumadine, there was 73% stenosis after lysis, and after three weeks the figure on average was the same. There was restenosis, but only very few patients had more than 20% improvement. If a big clot had been spontaneously lysed, this decrease would have been much more marked. These were therefore mainly organic stenoses. Sometimes there was a clot behind the stenosis but the majority were high grade organic stenoses. In another series in which the control was carried out after three days and after four weeks the same tendency was found. PTCA thus produces a significant improvement of stenosis.

We will now consider the end-diastolic volume index in the acute phase, after four weeks and after six months (Fig. 5a). The figure refers to a small group we controlled angiographically after six months. In the group without PTCA the left ventricle was enlarged, probably because the ischemic area was insufficiently reperfused and the myocardium was not functioning well. There are some patients with clear insufficiencies. In the group with PTCA the end-diastolic volume index was unchanged. With regard to the global ejection fraction, this remained more or less stable in the group without PTCA, while in the group with PTCA an improvement was found after four weeks (Fig. 5b). Between four weeks and six months there is no significant difference.

As has already been reported by several authors, the global ejection fraction does not give enough information. Figure 6a shows the wall motion of the angiogram in patients with anterior wall infarctions without PTCA. In the acute phase there is a large akinetic zone in the anterior wall: after four weeks it has improved a little, but at six months it has not changed any further. The hyperkinetic zone in the contralateral part can also be seen. In Fig. 6b, the group with PTCA, there is also a large

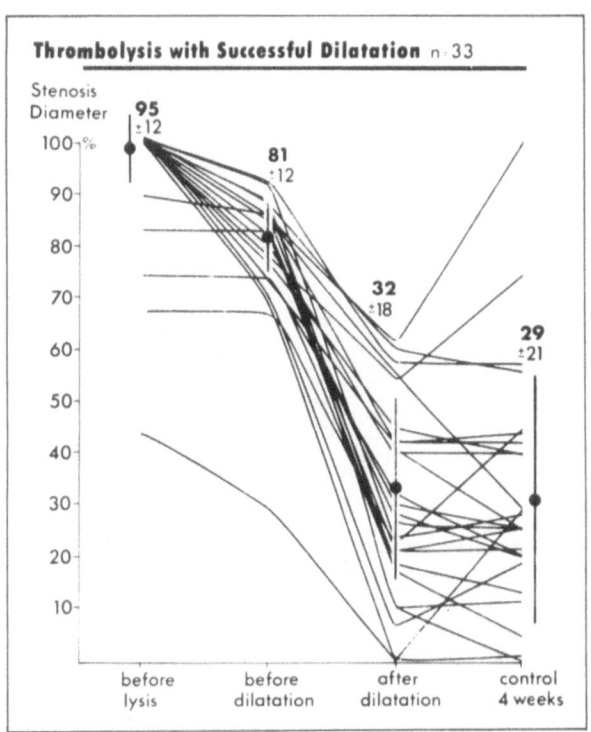

Fig. 4a. Development of coronary stenoses (diameter method) before lysis, before dilatation, after dilatation and after four weeks

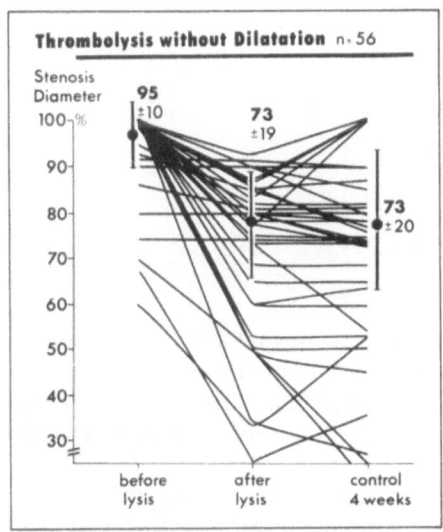

Fig. 4b. Development of coronary stenoses, thrombolysis without dilatation, before and after lysis and at the control study

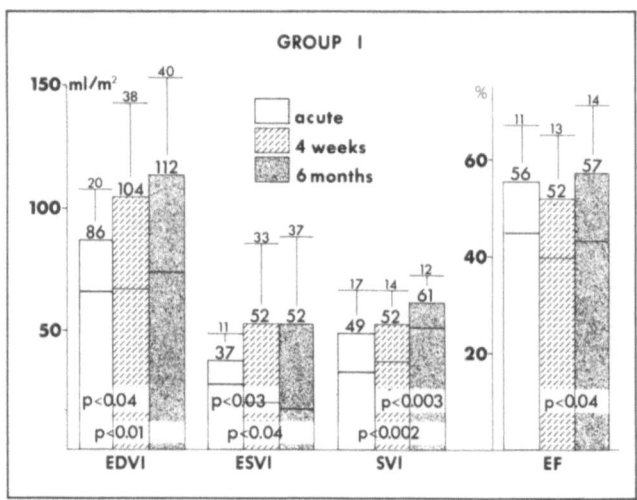

Fig. 5 a. Analysis of ventricular volume in thrombolysis without PTCA. EDVI: end-diastolic volume index; ESVI: end-systolic volume index; SVI: stroke volume index; EF: ejection fraction

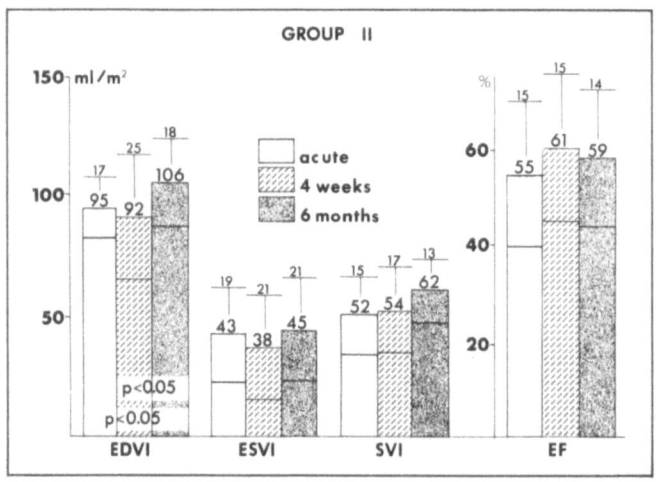

Fig. 5 b. Analysis of ventricular volume in thrombolysis with PTCA

hypokinesis to be seen, but after four weeks it is nearly normal and there is no significant additional improvement after six months. So the major change is already found after four weeks and there is not much improvement within the next few months. Thrombolysis shows better recovery of the wall motion with than without PTCA.

In conclusion, it seems to be feasible to perform PTCA, at least in single vessel disease, and sometimes also in double vessel disease immediately after thrombolysis. The preliminary results show that this is beneficial for the patient in terms of improvement of myocardial function, prevention of reinfarction, and in some cases of

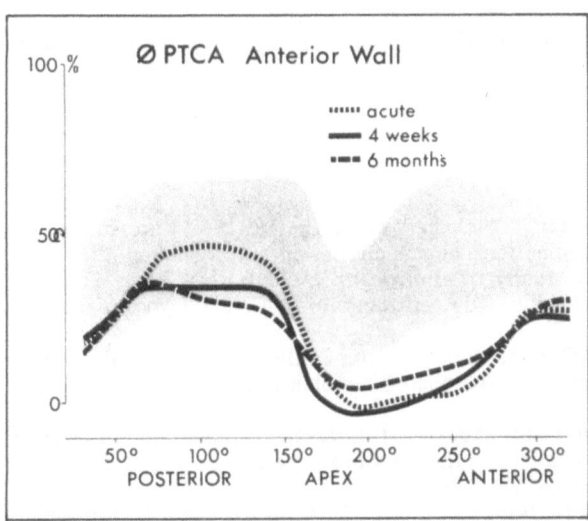

Fig. 6a. Segmental wall analysis in anterior wall infarction. Acute phase, control after four weeks and six months. Thrombolysis without PTCA

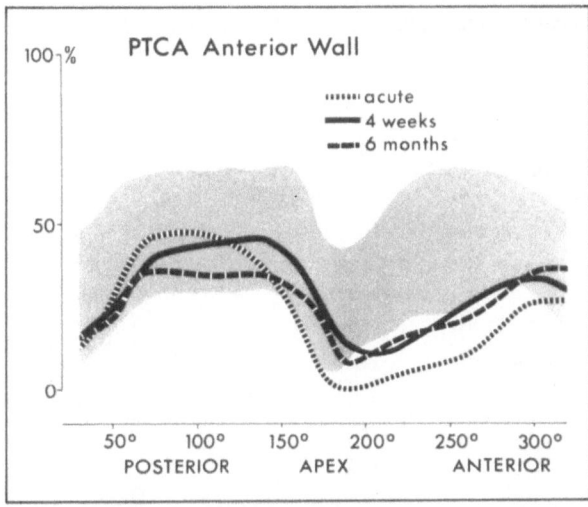

Fig. 6b. Segmental wall analysis in anterior wall infarction. Acute phase, control after four weeks and six months. Thrombolysis with PTCA

cardiac death (7–10). However, at present the numbers in our studies are not sufficient to produce significant data.

References

1. Collen D, Stump D, Van de Werf F, Jang I, Nobuhara M, Lijnen HR (1985) Coronary thrombolysis in dogs with intravenously administered human pro-urokinase. Circulation 72:384–388
2. DeWood MA, Spores J, Notske R, Mouser LT, Burroughs R, Golden MS, Lang HT (1980) Prevalence of total coronary occlusion during the early hours of transmural myocardial infarction. N Engl J Med 303:897–902
3. von Essen R, Uebis R, Schmidt W, Dörr R, Merx W, Meyer J, Effert S, Schweizer P, Erbel R, Bardos P, Minale C, Messmer BJ (1985) Intrakoronare Streptokinase beim akuten Herzinfarkt. Dtsch med Wschr 110:570–575
4. Harrison DG, Ferguson DW, Collins SM, Skorton DJ, Ericksen EE, Kioschos JM, Marcus ML, White CW (1984) Rethrombosis after reperfusion with streptokinase – Importance of geometry of residual lesions. Circulation 69:991–999
5. Mathey DG, Schofer J, Sheehan FH, Becker H, Tilsner V, Dodge HT (1985) Intravenous urokinase in acute myocardial infarction. Am J Cardiol 55:878–882
6. Meyer J, Merx W, Erbel R, Kiesslich T, Dörr R, Lambertz H, Bethge C, Krebs W, Bardos P, Minale C, Messmer BJ, Effert S (1982) Percutaneous transluminal coronary angioplasty immediately after intracoronary streptolysis of transmural myocardial infarction. Circulation 66:905–913
7. Rentrop P, Blanke H, Karsch KR, Wiegand V, Köstering H, Rahlf G, Oster H, Leitz K (1979) Wiedereröffnung des Infarktgefäßes durch transluminale Rekanalisation und intrakoronare Streptokinase-Applikation. Dtsch med Wschr 104:1438–1440
8. Serruys PW, Wijns W, Van den Brand M (1983) Is transluminal coronary angioplasty mandatory after successful thrombolysis? Quantitative coronary angiographic study. Br Heart J 50:257–265
9. Simoons ML, Serruys PW, Van den Brand M et al (1985) Improved survival after early thrombolysis in acute myocardial infarction. A randomized trial by the Interuniversity Cardiology Institute in The Netherlands. Lancet I:578–581
10. Van de Werf F, Ludbrook PA, Bergmann SR, Tiefenbrunn AJ, Fox KAA, de Geest H, Verstraete M, Collen D, Sobel BE (1984) Coronary thrombolysis with tissue-type plasminogen activator in patients with evolving myocardial infarction. N Engl J Med 310:609–613

Authors' address:
Prof. Dr. med. J. Meyer
Leiter der II. Medizinischen Klinik und Poliklinik
Klinikum der Johannes Gutenberg-Universität
Langenbeckstraße 1,
6500 Mainz
West Germany

Discussion

SIMOONS:

With regard to your data on the improvement of ejection fraction after PTCA, the lack of further distension of the ventricle, and the global data, were they referring to the two groups as you defined them at the outset, or were they the successful PTCA compared to those with whom it was not feasible?

MEYER:

These are the successful PTCAs versus the patients without PTCA. This is only a small study with 20 patients in the group without PTCA and 16 in the group with PTCA, since after six months it is very difficult to obtain the patients for a second time. Therefore the significance is also border-line.

MARGOLIS:

Do you think that the relatively poor success rate was related only to the complexity of the lesion or the fact that you were doing it in an acute setting? Perhaps if you had done these difficult lesions electively you might have been able to do them better?

MEYER:

No, I do not think so. I think the problem is that the lesions are difficult and also, a great number are included from our first study performed in 1982 when skill, apparatus and persistence were not as good as they are now. The question of when the PTCA is carried out, morning or night, is not important. I think the success rate can be improved. If we include the data from last year, with the steerable guides, the rate improves to about 75%. But it does not reach 90 or 93% as we have attained in stable or unstable angina because on average the patients are ten years older and the vessels more severely diseased than our stable and unstable angina patients.

Question:

Did you proceed to do PTCA in cases who did not open after streptokinase, and what were the results?

MEYER:

Where we were not able to open with streptokinase we used a special reopening catheter which was designed by Dr. Erbel. It is not a balloon catheter but a 3F catheter which goes via a normal 7F Cordis catheter. We use this very small infusion catheter just to make a hole in the thrombus, then pull it back and infuse streptokinase immediately in front of the thrombus. In some cases which are not included, where we have main stem arteries in the occlusion, we do not wait. We immediately go in with the balloon. If they are an emergency then we immediately open up.

Panel Discussion

Chairmen: W. Bleifeld and J. Van de Loo

Summary

The first part of the panel discussion deals with problems of early reocclusion of vessels after percutaneous coronary angioplasty (PTCA) or bypass surgery (CABG). Most investigators think that acute use of PTCA without thrombolytic therapy (e.g. streptokinase) will lead to high reocclusion rates. It is suspected that after PTCA substantial residual clot may still be present in the vessel.

A high risk of thrombus formation is expected if PTCA is performed in patients with unstable angina.

It is pointed out that at the site of reocclusion after PTCA atheroma, thrombus and bleeding in the vessel wall coexist. The role of the wall hematoma in reocclusion is not yet clear. A hematoma is most likely if the dilatation balloon is not imprinted at low pressures. In such cases over-inflation of the balloon is recommended.

The role of streptokinase in the prevention of reocclusion is discussed intensively. Some participants of the panel point out that the manner of application is of outstanding importance. Streptokinase administered directly into the coronary artery cannot maintain active concentrations at the site of occlusion over time. With regard to continuous drug administration the intravenous route is preferred.

Some investigators expressed their hope that in future new thrombolytic or platelet aggregation inhibiting drugs which can be given by the oral route will be developed. The interest focuses on prostacyclin-like drugs, Iloprost and drugs which increase cyclic AMP level in platelets.

After PTCA and CABG prevention of reocclusion is achieved by intravenous heparin (1000 units per hour) for 72 h, followed by coumarin or aspirin.

VAN DE LOO:

Reocclusion after surgery and PTCA Our first subject is the frequency of reocclusion, both after PTCA and surgery. Various figures have been quoted, but quite low, both after surgery and after PTCA. Has anyone found substantially different results or complications concerning the reocclusion rate?

ABLET

PTCA + streptokinase = low reocclusion rate We find that the acute use of PTCA without streptokinase leads to a high reocclusion rate. However, when PTCA is performed after streptokinase administration, we have similar figures to those presented by the panel.

166

MEYER:

Residual clot = high reocclusion rate

This supports our findings that the rate of reocclusion is much higher if, after thrombolysis, there is substantial clot material still in the vessel, at the thrombus, and the same applies if only PTCA is performed immediately, without streptokinase. The thrombus is compressed, and there is enough thrombotic material to be the nucleus of a very early reocclusion.

ABLET:

PTCA/ unstable angina

We also find a similar situation when PTCA is performed in patients with unstable angina, and who do not have an obvious thrombus. We have come to believe that the arterial wall in patients with unstable angina is very different from that in patients with stable angina.

MEYER:

We have a large series of cases of stable and unstable angina, but we do not have a higher rate of complications, i.e. immediate reocclusion in the unstable versus the stable angina patient. However, a higher rate of reoccurrence of the stenosis does occur after six months.

HOCH:

At the site of occlusion we have three main situations: a thrombus, atheroma, and bleeding in the vessel wall. We have spoken about thrombolysis and we are able to prevent reocclusion. We can perform PTCA to dilate the stenosis, but my question is: what is the role of hematoma in preventing reocclusion?

Question:

Hematoma of vessel wall

It is very difficult to prove the presence of a hematoma. Autopsy of patients who had died after acute myocardial infarction revealed no significant bleeding which may have caused an occlusion. There is a hematoma in the atheroma, but it is impossible to find in vivo, and in the cases autopsied they did not play an important role. There is no doubt, though, that hematoma may contribute in some cases.

MARGOLIS:

We have developed criteria for a group of patients who we think have a slight rupture, with wall hematoma. We generally perform PTCA as early as possible. If a catheter is set up early enough, we

167

sometimes do not give streptokinase at all. If there is no imprint of the stenosis on the balloon at low pressure, we highly suspect that this is a plaque rupture with wall hematoma. These seem to be the same patients who have a tendency to reocclusion, but they do respond to over-inflation of the balloon. Prolonged over-inflation of the balloon results in the artery remaining open.

MEYER:

In my view, there is no difference between a wall hematoma and a fresh thrombus, because both are weak materials. How can an acute hematoma and a fresh thrombus be dinstinguished?

GANZ:

I think that the pathologists agree that the hematoma is a secondary phenomenon, i.e. an ulceration of the plaque, and not a rupture.

VAN DE LOO:

Since there are no substantially different opinions on the magnitude of the reocclusion rate, we may conclude that most of those present have corresponding figures for reocclusion during surgery and after PTCA.

BLEIFELD:

Duration of streptokinase treatment

We have heard that the length of the stenosis decreases from the first to the third day, and that a residual thrombus remains. Would prolongation of thrombolysis be effective? Are there any animal experiments showing reocclusion rates with different duration of streptokinase treatment?

LUCCHESI:

We have only studied streptokinase at 30 and 90 min after total occlusion. The same degree of efficacy with respect to revascularization occurred. So the duration of the thrombosis over that period of time does not seem to alter the efficacy of streptokinase, nor does is it seem to change the patterns of reflow. Ultimately, reocclusion recurs in all cases.

BLEIFELD:

Was there a residual thrombus in the animals that were treated for 90 min and then had a reocclusion?

LUCCHESI:

Yes, there was.

BLEIFELD:

Is there any evidence from angiographic data or other clinical data that thrombolysis should be prolonged?

VERSTRAETE:

There appears to be no evidence as yet; further experimentation is required.

BLEIFELD:

It may be that the angiographic data are misused, because even an 80% reduction in diameter of stenosis would mean a reduction of cross-sectional area of 95%. Under any experimental conditions, a reduction in the cross-section of the vessel above 85–90% will result in total disappearance of wall motion and wall thickness. Thus, if the diameter of the stenosis in a patient is still 80–85% after thrombolysis, we should proceed with angioplasty.

UEBIS:

The data from the time immediately after lysis to the 3rd day, and the data from follow-up after the second or third week, may show that there is not very much residual thrombus within those stenoses, because otherwise there should be another decrease after the 3rd day. About 5–7 patients (i.e. less than 10%) showed angiographic evidence of residual thrombus. It should be remembered that we are comparing data after i.c. thrombolysis with data after i.v. thrombolysis, and there may be some difference.

VERSTRAETE:

A diameter of stenosis of 80% on a vessel of 3 mm results in a residual lumen of 0.6 mm. The smallest guide wire is 0.5 mm. The theoretical drop in pressure across this lesion is so large that there is no driving pressure in the distal part of the stenosis. Although the angiographic system is not very effective in evaluating the coronary stenosis, I am certain that the lesions are not so severe.

LUCCHESI:

Intracoronary and intravenous streptokinase

There is a difference between i.c. streptokinase and i.v. streptokinase. With i.c. streptokinase it is very difficult to maintain a thrombolytic concentration of streptokinase at the site. On the other hand, if you achieve a systemic effect, you are more likely to prevent that thrombus reforming. In our experimental model we purposely limited the streptokinase to the site of the thrombus. It was most disappointing to see re-formation of the thrombus occur so rapidly. However, if we had a systemic lytic effect, we would extent that time in which rethrombosis occurs. Therefore I think that we have to analyse the study very carefully on the basis of whether it is an intracoronary or an intravenous study.

BLEIFELD:

PTCA – promptly or delayed?

This leads us to the question of when angioplasty should be performed – promptly, or one day later?

MEYER:

We began with immediate PTCA treatment, but there was always the question of why it should not be delayed to the next day. We do not know which stenosis will reocclude and we are not certain whether heparin or coumarin will keep the vessel open. With this uncertainty we have no choice but to perform PTCA immediately, if possible. An area of stenosis of 95% means that the myocardium is still underperfused, and a reduction of stenosis to 30% or 40% results in a normal flow. These are the two reasons why we perform PTCA immediately. If this high grade stenosis is maintained for 24 h, you still have the stunned myocardium. These are very important points. I know there are practical difficulties in 24 h treatment, but maintenance of therapy is vital.

VAN DE WERF:

Reocclusion – the role of heparin and prostacyclin

Dr. Lucchesi, you have advised the use of heparin and prostacyclin in the prevention of reocclusion. However, you cannot give these drugs orally, so I would like to hear what you advise for long-term treatment.

LUCCHESI:

In the future you will be able to give prostacyclin-like compounds orally. We now know that the amount of prostacyclin necessary to inhibit platelet function is very small, much smaller than is needed to achieve a hemodynamic effect. Heparin, unfortunately, is still a

170

problem with respect to oral administration, but you do not need heparin in the presence of prostacyclin. In fact, you could use prostacyclin in a patient undergoing cardiopulmonary bypass and you can circumvent the use of heparin. Prostacyclin is quite effective as an antithrombotic agent.

VAN DE WERF:

Can one use aspirin as in Dr. Folze's experiments with dogs?

LUCCHESI:

Aspirin does not prevent thrombosis in vivo

The aspirin story is quite complex, which is why I pointed out that the Folze model may be misinterpreted. In our model for instance, where we have endothelial injury and the growth of the thrombus, aspirin is completely ineffective. It is possible that we have not been administering the correct dose. An excessive dose of aspirin is worse or less effective than using nothing at all; perhaps a very low dose of aspirin is needed. Furthermore while aspirin will inhibit platelet aggregation in vitro it certainly does not prevent coronary thrombosis in vivo. Dr. Folze's model is looking at an entirely different problem, not at a thrombus.

VERSTRAETE:

Dr. Lucchesi, when you were inducing your experimental thrombosis, the animals were flooded by prostacyclin. This is unrealistic, however, because the topic that you discussed was rethrombosis. Therefore, if you wanted to mimic our aim, avoiding a rethrombosis in a damaged vessel, you should make the thrombosis first, lyse it, and then induce a second thrombosis under the protection of prostacyclin. Did you obtain a hypotensive effect with the massive doses of prostacyclin that you used?

LUCCHESI:

Role of prostacyclin in preventing reocclusion

I carried out two different kinds of studies. In one, prostacyclin was given before mechanical occlusion of the coronary vessel. Here we were interested in looking at salvage of reperfused myocardium, and myocardium was indeed salvaged. The second study was looking at thrombolysis, after which we gave streptokinase, followed by prostacyclin. In other words it mimicked the clinical situation as closely as possible. We gave prostacyclin in pharmacological doses that produced a very severe hemodynamic effect. Then we reduced the dose of prostacyclin to the point where it was ineffective as an antithrombolytic agent. But when we combined this with aminophylline, we now had an effect. I therefore suggest that it is possible to

171

give prostacyclin in a dose that does not produce hemodynamic consequences, and yet achieve one's goal. It is interesting that if you take platelets that have been exposed to prostacyclin in vivo, and the prostacyclin treatment is discontinued, thus allowing all the hemodynamics to return, an hour later they still fail to aggregate to arachidonic acid, collagen and ATP. So the prostacyclin effect is very long-lived and we now have to return to the laboratory and work out the pharmacokinetics of prostacyclin and prostacyclin-like compounds to find an effective dose that does not produce the hemodynamic effect.

GANZ:

In my experience you can do that for a couple of hours but not for days. We want to cover at least four of five days to avoid rethrombosis.

LUCCHESI:

I agree with you. Prostacyclin is a very difficult drug to use, so I would suggest paying more attention to drugs like Iloprost and there are many other derivatives of prostacyclin which are being developed, some of which are orally effective. I have a lot of hope for the future.

Question:

When we discussed this problem at the AGA meetings the group from Rochester presented its data on PTCA, and they could not find this good effect. They found the same amount of thrombus at the endothelial lesion, with and without prostacyclin. Could you comment on this? And the second thing is, the encouraging data on prostacyclin in cardiopulmonary bypass in England could not be repeated by the Boston group. Could you please comment on this too?

LUCCHESI:

I think we are talking about different kinds of studies, the facts of which are not at present clearly in my mind.

GANZ:

Prostacyclin – mechanism of action

We have used your Salazar model of thrombosis but find it has a problem in that you are blurring everything. When you apply prostacyclin you dilate the arterioles, you produce an afterload reducing effect that may make your heart smaller, and contraction better. It may be an indirect, extramyocardial effect. Were you aware of these potential traps?

LUCCHESI:

The Salazar model is like a hundred and twenty volts compared to the microamps we are using. All we do is to injure the endothelium, as we know from histological studies. We then discontinue the current and the thrombus forms naturally. I think prostacyclin will not be used in the future. We are now looking at a number of drugs which increase cyclic AMP specifically in platelets, and these are chemically derived compounds which can be given orally, intravenously, or in any other way. I am studying prostacyclin to determine its mechanism of action. If I can determine the mechanism then I will look for other mechanisms, other therapeutic interventions that will reproduce the same effect and hopefully the outcome will be the same.

VAN DE LOO:

Current anti-thrombotic treatment schedules The first three speakers talked about antithrombotic procedures after the intervention, but did not inform us about their exact treatment schedule. Dr. Uebis, you said that patients were under coumarin. Did you use coumarin alone, or did you begin with heparin? And on which drug did you consider your patients were under effective anticoagulation?

UEBIS:

At the time of the first control angiogram on the third day, patients were under heparin alone, at a dosage of 1000 units per hour. That means at the time of the control angiogram patients were either on coumarin or aspirin. There was no clear regimen to divide patients, no randomization, for instance, but every patient had some form of anticoagulation, either the coumarin or aspirin.

VAN DE LOO:

And the heparin was the standard dose, 1000 units per hour, irrespective of laboratory results?

UEBIS:

Yes, because of the difficulty of having double parameters to check.

173

MEYER:

We have patients on heparin for the first 72 h but it is not given routinely, we check every four to six hours and always have prolongation between 80–120 s. Patients are only heparinized according to the values obtained and then overlapping, they receive coumarin, and only until the coumarin value (the Quick value) is between 15 and 25 then the heparin is stopped. Otherwise we have the overlap. We try to have a really strict anticoagulation system which is always controlled four times in 24 h. But we also have the problem that sometimes during the night the laboratory gives a value that is not safe and then we have to change; you know all these problems. But we try really hard to have patients controlled at four or six hour intervals.

MESSMER:

We welcome patients with a high dose of heparin since it is short-acting and does not really disturb surgery, but too much aspirin is not liked because it is a long-acting agent. After surgery, the problem of reocclusion of the stenosis is resolved, but nevertheless as a rule we keep all our patients who undergo coronary bypass surgery on anti-coagulants (on coumarin) for four to six months. I know that this is open to discussion. Generally, if you have patients with bad run-off, with a bad peripheral vascular bed, it is better to have them on anticoagulants. When a great deal of coronary artery surgery is performed, it is better to have four to six months.

Clinical experience with rt-PA
in the Cooperative European Trials
1. rt-PA versus placebo

D. P. de Bono

Department of Cardiology, The Royal Infirmary, Edinburgh, Scotland (U.K.)

Human recombinant tissue type plasminogen activator (rt-PA) first became available in Europe for medium-scale clinical trials in acute myocardial infarction early in 1984, provided by Boehringer Ingelheim GmbH in collaboration with Genentech Inc. A small steering committee was set up under the chairmanship of Professor M. Verstraete to plan and coordinate these trials – the members of this committee, and of the others who participated in the studies, are listed at the end of this paper. On the basis of experience with previous thrombolysis trials using other agents (1, 5) and of pilot studies with rt-PA in Europe and the United States of America (2, 4), it was decided that the first priority was to establish whether rt-PA was going to be an effective, rapid and safe thrombolytic agent when given by the intravenous route.

Design of first-phase European trials

Because we were anxious to initiate thrombolytic therapy as soon as possible after presentation of the patient, we decided to forego preliminary angiography to confirm occlusion of the presumed infarct-related vessel. Coronary patency was assessed by angiography 90 minutes after the start of treatment, and we set up two studies, one to compare coronary patency in patients given rt-PA versus placebo, and the other to compare coronary patency after rt-PA with patency after the "best available regime" of intravenous streptokinase (Table 1). Professor Rutsch will be describing the rt-PA versus streptokinase study in the following paper. The initial results of both studies have already been published (6, 7).

rt-PA versus placebo in acute myocardial infarction

The *entry criteria* for this study are summarised in Table 2. It should be noted that the ECG criteria for inclusion are more stringent than in a number of other trials – from previous experience we anticipated that approximately 80% of patients fulfilling these criteria would have an occluded infarct-related vessel at angiography 90 minutes later. *Exclusion criteria* were age below 20 or over 70, previous myocardial infarction (to assist identification of the infarct related vessel) and the usual contraindications to thrombolytic therapy (Table 3). All patients gave their consent to participation in a form acceptable to local Ethics of Medical Research committees. Patients who still had an occluded vessel at 90 minutes were able to receive intracoronary streptokinase or undergo mechanical thrombus perforation plus coronary angioplasty at the discretion of their physician.

Table 1. Plan of first-phase European trials of rt-PA in acute myocardial infarction

FIRST PHASE EUROPEAN TPA TRIALS
(1984–1985)

1ST ACUTE INFARCTION
Duration < 6 hours, clinical & ECG criteria
NO pretreatment angiography

TPA vs. streptokinase   TPA vs. placebo
(7 centres)   (6 centres)
Random allocation   Random allocation
to I/V TPA or SK   to I/V TPA or placebo

Angiography at 90 minutes

Angiograms assessed "blind"

End-points: Angiographic patency
Haemostatic measurements
Complications

Table 2. Entry criteria for the rt-PA versus placebo study

1. Age 20 to 70.
2. History of typical ischaemic chest pain lasting for more than 30 minutes; onset of pain not more than 6 hours before start of treatment.
3. Typical ECG changes: ST elevation (60 msec after J point) of 2 mm or more in at least 2 standard frontal plane leads or 3 mm or more in at least two precordial leads. Q waves not required and did not exclude.
4. Absence of exclusion criteria.

Table 3. Exclusion criteria for the rt-PA versus placebo study

1. Cardiogenic shock
2. Usual contraindictions to thrombolytic therapy:
   Prolonged or traumatic cardiac massage;
   Pregnant or currently menstruating;
   Previous streptokinase therapy;
   Oral anticoagulants;
   Recent head injury;
   Recent (6 weeks) major surgery;
   Recent (3 months) gastric bleeding;
   Recent (3 months) urinary tract bleeding;
   Previous CVA;
   Diabetic proliferative retinopathy;
   Known cancer, renal or hepatic disease;
   Alcohol or drug abuse
3. Previous myocardial infarction
4. Onset of severe pain more than 6 hours before start of treatment
5. Anticipated problems with follow-up

176

Treatment

Patients were given routine treatment for pain relief. As soon as possible after admission blood was drawn for enzyme and coagulation studies, a bolus injection of 5000 i.u. of heparin was given intravenously, and patients randomly allocated to receive either rt-PA (0.75 mg per kg body weight) or placebo by intravenous infusion over 90 minutes. The rt-PA and placebo were identically packaged and indistinguishable in appearance. Randomization was by telephone call to a central office. Coronary angiograms were performed 90 minutes after the start of the infusion, and recorded on 35 mm cine film.

End-points

The *primary end-points* of the study were:
1) Coronary patency assessed by angiography 90 minutes after the start of infusion of rt-PA or placebo.
2) Clinical outcome and complications.
3) Changes in haemostatic function, in particular fibrinogen and fibrinogen degradation products.
Coronary patency was assessed by a group of observers independent of any of the participating centres, who reviewed the coronary arteriograms without knowledge of the treatment given. At least three views of the left coronary artery and two of the right coronary artery were required. Coronary arteriograms were reported segment by segment using a semiquantitative scoring system (Table 4). Patients were regarded as having "anterior" infarcts if there was 2 mm or more of ST elevation in leads V2, V3 or V4, and "non anterior" infarcts if the ST elevation was in other leads. Infarct related vessels were regarded as "patent" if there was no stenosis greater than grade 3 in the territory of the infarct related vessel (left anterior descending coronary artery for anterior, right or circumflex coronary arteries for "non-anterior" infarcts), and "occluded" if there was a stenosis of grade 4 or 5. It should be noted that this is a fundamentally different form of assessment from that used in the "TIMI" trial (3) where assessment was on the basis of the degree of perfusion of a vessel previously shown to be occluded. Assessment was based on the first technically satisfactory injection of the angiogram, to avoid the possibility that patency was resulting from the action of coronary injection rather than the thrombolytic drug.
Methods for measuring plasma fibrinogen and fibrinogen degradation products are referenced in the "Lancet" reports.

Table 4. Scoring criteria in assessment of the 90 minute coronary arteriogram

0	Normal vessel
1	Stenosis < 50 % diameter
2	Stenosis > 50 %, < 90 % diameter
3	Stenosis > 90 %, but distal vessel fills completely within 3 cardiac cycles
4	Stenosis > 90 % without complete filling of distal vessel
5	Occluded

Grades 0 to 3 classed as patent, grades 4 & 5 occluded

Table 5. Baseline characteristics of patients on admission

		rt-PA group n = 64	Placebo group n = 65
Male/female		59/5	59/6
Age (yr)	Median	56.4	54.9
	Range	(32–67)	(26–70)
Duration from onset of pain to start of infusion		3.4 (1.2–5.8)	3.3 (1.0–6.0)
Anterior MI		31/63	31/65
Systolic BP:	Median	130	130
	Range	(90–200)	(100–180
Pulmonary crepitations		14/63	10/65

Table 6. Coronary patency at 90 minutes in the rt-PA versus placebo study

	TPA/Placebo 127 Patients	
	63 TPA	64 Placebo
Patent	38 (61.3%)	13 (21%)
Occluded	24	48
Not assessable	0	2
Not available	1	1
	Placebo	rt-PA
Patients with occluded vessels	49	24
Treated with SK or UK	21	6
Patent after SK or UK	12	5
Immediate PTCA ± SK	8	2

Table 7. Clinical events during hospital stay in rt-PA versus placebo study

	rt-PA	Placebo
Fall of blood pressure to < 90 mm syst.	7	7
Cardiogenic shock	1	2
Pulmonary oedema	2	3
Bradycardia < 50 beats/min	9	4
AV block	2	4
Atrial fibrillation	3	6
Accelerated idioventricular rhythm	11	12
Ventricular tachycardia	12	11
Ventricular fibrillation	2	3
Pericarditis	3	4
Exacertion of chest pain	10	10
Deinite reinfarction	3	0
Signs of bleeding	11	5
Blood transfusion	0	1
None of the above	23	26
Mortality	1	4

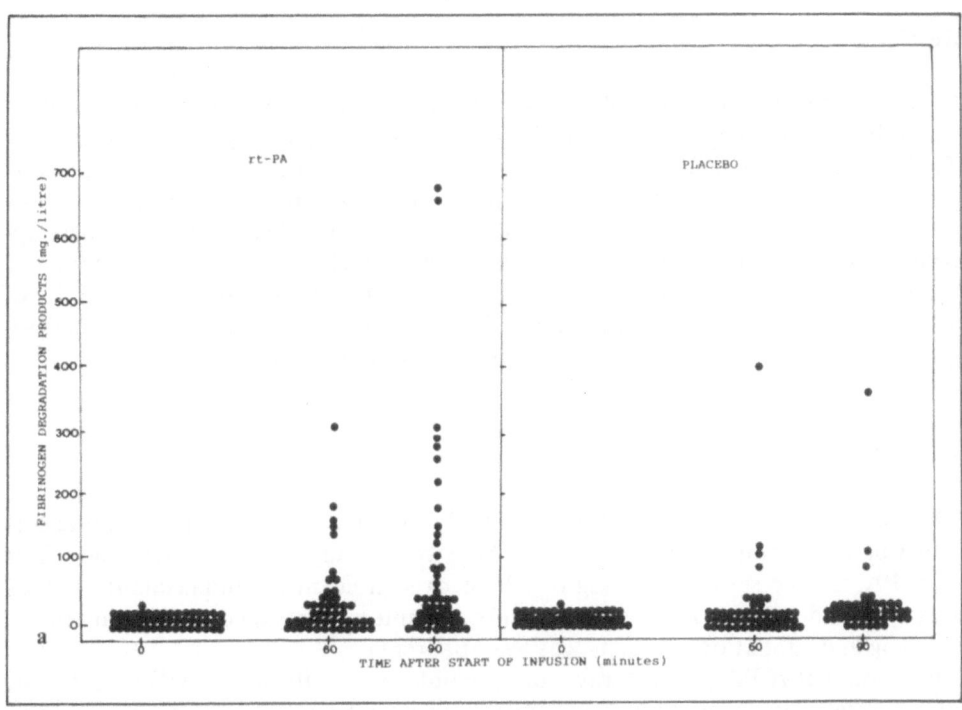

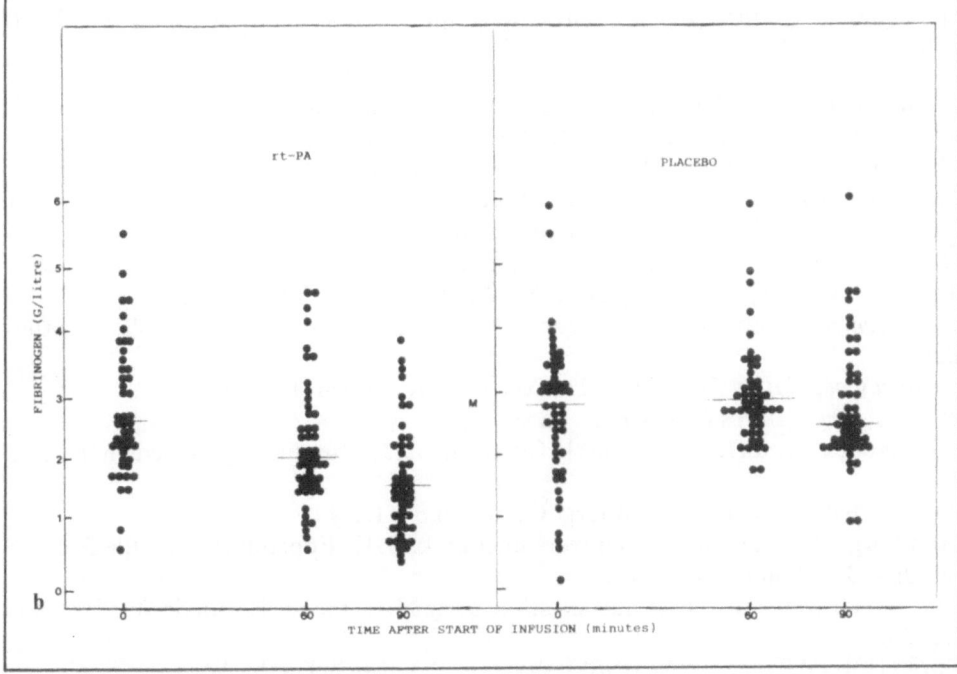

Fig. 1. Plasma concentration of fibrinogen (a) and fibrinogen (b) degradation products before, and 60 and 90 minutes after, the start of infusion of rt-PA or placebo.

Results

Patients in the placebo and rt-PA groups were comparable in age, sex distribution, site of infarct and length of history (Table 5). Coronary patency results are given in Table 6. 62% of patients in the rt-PA group, and 21% of patients in the placebo group had patent vessels at 90 minutes (p < 0.0001). Numbers are too small to show any significant effect on mortality. Clinical events are detailed in Table 7 – there appeared to be no significant adverse haemodynamic effects of rt-PA infusion, and there were no major bleeding problems, although minor haematomas at the site of arterial puncture were more common in the TPA group. The results of plasma fibrinogen and fibrinogen degradation product estimations are given in Fig. 1.

Discussion

The use of rt-PA was associated with a highly significant increase in 90 minute coronary patency compared with placebo. There were no adverse haemodynamic effects of rt-PA, and no serious bleeding problems. A significant fall in plasma fibrinogen was observed in the rt-PA treated patients, but interestingly a corresponding rise in fibrinogen degradation products was less apparent.

The hope that rt-PA given intravenously would be an effective, easy and safe way of securing early coronary patency appears to have been fulfilled. It remains to be seen whether the vessels remain patient, and whether effective thrombolysis is responsible for improved left ventricular function and reduced mortality. These aspects will be the subject of future trials.

Acknowledgements. The Trial was conducted by the European cooperative study group for recombinant human tissue-type plasminogen activator:
Steering Committee Prof. M. Verstraete (Leuven) (Chairman); R. J. Lennane (Ingleheim) (Clinical Coordinator); D. P. de Bono (Edinburgh); J. Lubsen (Rotterdam); D. Mathey (Hamburg); R. von Essen (Aachen).
Advisory Board J. Hampton (Nottingham), H. J. Jesdinsky (Düsseldorf), D. G. Julian (Newcastle), W. Shaper (Bad Nauheim), L. Wilhelmsen (Göteborg).
Data Centre J. Lubsen, R. W. Brower, P. Fioretti, B. Soward, M. Bokslag (Rotterdam).
Central Coagulation Laboratory D. Collen, H. R. Lijnen (Leuven).
Participating Centres (rt-PA/placebo study).
Amsterdam: Academisch Medisch Centrum: A. J. Dunning, G. Hoedemaker, K. Romyn
The Hague: Ziekenhuis Leyenburg: G. A. van der Kley
Hamburg: 2. Medizinische Universitätsklinik, UK Eppendorf: W. Bleifeld, D. Mathey, J. Schofer
Leuven: Universitair Ziekenhuis Gasthuisberg: H. de Geest, F. van de Werf, J. Vanhaecke
Paris: Hôpital Tenon: J. Acar, A. Vahanian, P. L. Michel, J. M. Weber
Tours: Centre Hospitalier Regional et Universitaire: M. Brochier, Ph. Raynaud, B. Charbonnier

References

1. Been M, de Bono DP, Muir AL, Boulton FE, Hillis WS, Hornung R (1985) Coronary thrombolysis with intravenous anisoylated plasminogen streptokinase complex. Br Heart J 53:253–259
2. Collen D, Topol EJ, Tiefenbrunn AJ et al (1984) Coronary thrombolysis with recombinant human tissue-type plasminogen activator: a prospective, randomized, placebo controlled trial. Circulation 70:1012–1017
3. The TIMI study group (1985) The thrombolysis in myocardial infarction (TIMI) trial. Phase 1 findings. New Engl J Med 312:932–936
4. van der Werf F, Ludbrook PA, Bergmann SR et al (1984) Coronary thrombolysis with tissue-type plasminogen activator in patients with evolving myocardial infarction. New Engl J Med 310:609–613
5. Verstraete M, van der Loo J, Jesdinsky HJ (1980) Streptokinase in myocardial infarction – extended report of the European cooperative trial. Acta Med Scand 68 (Suppl):1–55
6. Verstraete M, Bernard R, Bory M et al (1985) Randomized trial of intravenous recombinant tissue-type plasminogen activator versus intravenous streptokinase in acute myocardial infarction. Report from the European cooperative study group. Lancet i:842–847
7. Verstraete M, Bleifeld W, Brower RW et al (1985) Double blind randomised trial of intravenous tissue type plasminogen activator versus placebo in acute myocardial infarction. Lancet ii:965–969

Author's address:

D. P. de Bono, M.D., F.R.C.P. (Ed)
Department of Cardiology
The Royal Infirmary
Edinburgh EH3 9YW
Scotland (U.K.)

Clinical experience with rt-PA in the Cooperative European Trials 2. rt-PA versus streptokinase

W. Rutsch

Department of Cardiology, Klinikum Charlottenburg, Free University, Berlin

Introduction

Most of the randomised trials of intravenous streptokinase in acute coronary care have failed to achieve statistically significant changes in mortality and have failed to be generally convincing. The fear of hemorrhagic complications and less seriously, of pyrogenic and allergic reactions has limited extensive use of intravenous streptokinase as a thrombolytic agent in patients with acute myocardial infarction. This explains the keen interest in tissue-type plasminogen activator (rt-PA), a naturally occurring protein in man which has a greater clot selectivity than streptokinase and urokinase and which, at thrombolytic doses, has not induced systemic fibrinolysis in animals or in patients treated so far.

Clot selectivity appears to render t-PA useful for coronary thrombolysis in part because:

1. Clot lysis can be accomplished with t-PA in doses that do not induce a systemic lytic state characterised by consumption of alpha-2-antiplasmin, depletion of plasminogen, fibrinogenolysis, increased circulating fibrinogen degradation products and predisposition to systemic bleeding.
2. Definitive surgical treatment of high grade residual stenoses can be initiated promptly after successful thrombolysis with t-PA in contrast to conventional activators because of its short biological half-life of some minutes.
3. Bleeding from arterial puncture sites or from resuscitation may be less frequent because of the conspicuous anticoagulant effects of elevated FDPs and prolonged depletion of fibrinogen after infusion of streptokinase.

I should not only like to point out the potential advantages of clot selectivity but also to circumscribe the meaning of this term, emphasizing its relative rather than absolute nature.

Plasmin formed at the fibrin surface is capable of rapidly inducing clot lysis. Any plasmin escaping into the circulation is rapidly inactivated by alpha-2-antiplasmin. Fibrinolysis induced pharmacologically with streptokinase or urokinase results in conversion of circulating plasminogen to plasmin; consumption of alpha-2-antiplasmin, degradation of fibrinogen, plasminogen and impairment of systemic hemostasis. Fibrinolysis induced with t-PA resembles physiologically induced fibrinolysis much more than with conventional activators. The affinity of free, circulating t-PA for circulating plasminogen is low in contrast to the affinity for plasminogen when both are bound to fibrin in a thrombus. Thus plasmin does not accumulate in circulating plasma but is formed at the fibrin surface of the clot.

The aim of this single-blind randomised trial in 7 centres was to compare the relative effectiveness, in terms of angiographically proven coronary patency, of 2 intravenous drug regimens – heparin plus rt-PA versus heparin plus streptokinase. The safety of the 2 drug regimens was also compared, and their effect on components of the coagulation and fibrinolytic system assessed (2).

Methods

Patients between 21 and 70 years and without previous myocardial infarction were eligible for participation if severe chest pain typical of myocardial ischaemia persisted for at least 30 min. In addition, at least a 2 mm ST segment elevation (60 ms after J point) in 2 or more standard frontal leads or 3 mm in 2 or more precordial leads had to be present. All patients were randomised within 6 hours of the onset of pain. Patients were excluded if they met any of the following criteria: hypotension (systolic blood pressure below 90 mm Hg) and a heart rate over 110/min in a clinical setting typical of cardiogenic shock; history of previous infarction, cerebrovascular accident, major surgery during the previous 6 months; severe hypertension (over 200 mm Hg systolic blood pressure); prolonged or traumatic heart massage or artificial respiration; a known bleeding disorder; recent major trauma, major hepatic or renal disease, cancer; anticipated problems with heart catheterisation etc.

Computations done in the design phase showed that if 20% of the angiograms of each group (rt-PA and streptokinase) were scored as non-perfused the 95% confidence interval of the difference would range from − 15 to +15%, assuming a total study size of 120 patients. Thus, we aimed for a total of 120 patients, 60 allocated to rt-PA and 60 to streptokinase.

Patients randomised to the rt-PA group received a bolus injection of 5,000 IU heparin followed by rt-PA (0.75 mg/kg body weight) given by infusion pump over 90 min (Fig. 1), the dose of rt-PA was based on the results of a previous trial. The rt-PA was produced by expression of the cloned human t-PA gene in mammalian-cell culture.

The patients allocated to streptokinase treatment received an intravenous bolus injection of 5,000 IU heparin, 0.25 g methylprednisolone, and 0.5 g acetylsalicylic acid, followed by an infusion of 250 ml of 5% glucose containing 1.5 mill IU streptokinase given by infusion pump over 60 min; this dose was based on the experience of Schroeder et al. (1). Blood samples were collected for enzyme and coagulation studies before, 60 and 90 min after the start of the infusion.

Selective coronary angiography was done between 75 and 90 min after the start of the infusion of the thrombolytic drug. Coronary angiograms were evaluated by the independent angiography evaluation group and they represented the primary endpoint of the study. Each angiogram was read by 2 assessors from a panel of experienced cardiologists and radiologists independent of the participating units. They did not know which treatment the patient had received. Each assessor scored the arteriogram individually, and recorded the results of visual assessment with the use of a predetermined qualitative code: (0) normal vessel; (1) mild stenosis less than 50%; (2) moderate stenosis greater than 50% but less than 90%; (3) severe stenosis greater than 90%, but distal vessels fill completely, not through collaterals, with 3 cardiac cycles; (4) subtotal occlusion, distal vessel does not fill within 3 cardiac cycles; (5) total occlusion with or without collateral filling.

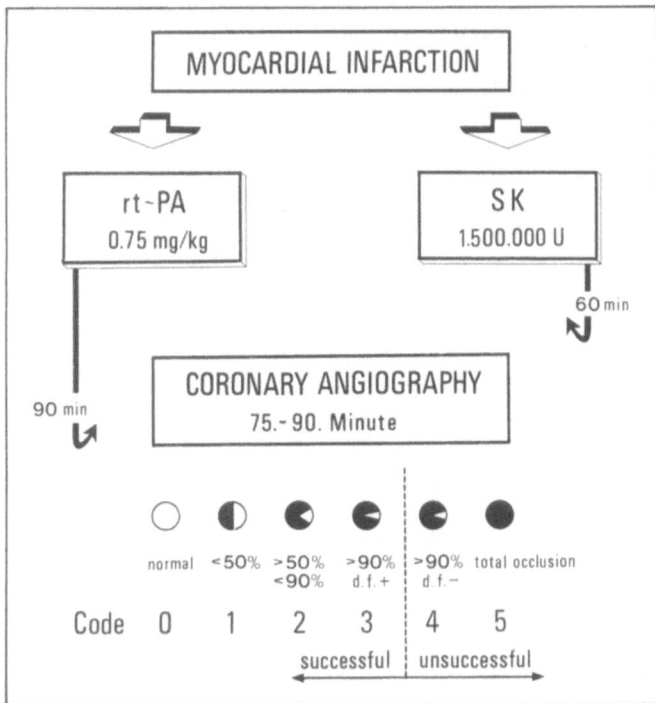

Fig. 1. Randomisation to tissue-type plasminogen activator or streptokinase; infusion time 90 min and 60 min respectively. Coronary angiography 75th–90th min after the start of infusion. Assessment of the angiograms with the use of a qualitative code (d.f.$+/-$: distal vessel fills completely or not within 3 cardiac cycles)

Pre-intervention angiography was not done in the present study, since we were anxious to start intravenous thrombolytic therapy as early as possible. The number of patients with initially patent or spontaneously reperfused vessels is thus unknown. Reperfusion in the context of the present trial is therefore a judgment based on the patency of vessels in the post-treatment angiogram, the appearance of vessels, in particular the knowledge of the presumed infarct-related vessel as determined by the electrocardiogram.

Successful reperfusion had probably occurred if all the vessels in the infarct-related area had scores of 3 or less and there were no "missing vessels". Reperfusion was assessed as unsuccessful if any of the vessels in the infarct-related area was seen as totally occluded (code 5) or a subtotally occluded vessel with poor distal filling (code 4).

Results

129 patients were randomised to the 2 treatment groups. Baseline characteristics are summarised in Table 1. In 1 patient the allotted streptokinase treatment could not be given because of shock. Cardiac catheterisation could not be done in 1 patient because both femoral arteries were severely stenotic. In the 128 patients who received

Table 1. Events after administration of infusion but before hospital discharge

	Duration first 48 h		3rd day until discharge	
	rt-PA	SK	rt-PA	SK
Bleeding at puncture site	3	10*	1	2
Haematoma at cath. site	12	19*	1	3
Blood transfusion given	2	4*	2	1
Hospital mortality	0	0	3	3
Angina pectoris	14*	5	8	12*
Reinfarction	0	1	2	3
Cardiogenic shock	1	1	1	1

Table 2. Selected baseline characteristics of patients on admission

	rt-PA n = 64	SK group n = 65
Males	52	54
Age (yr)	55 (32–70)	54 (37–70)
Time onset M1 to infusion	30 (1.1–5.5)	2.6 (0.8–5.9)
< 1 h	0	1
Between 1–2 h	14	9
2–3 h	16	26
3–4 h	22	19
4–5 h	7	7
5–6 h	4	1
uncertain	1	2

treatment there was no difference between the 2 treatment groups in terms of arrhythmia, blood pressure, heart rate, and allergic reactions. There was 1 transient ischaemic attack in the rt-PA group and a confirmed cerebrovascular accident in the streptokinase group. During the first 48 h haematoma and prolonged bleeding at puncture site were more frequently a problem in the streptokinase-treated patients, but blood transfusions were given infrequently in both groups (Table 2).

Figure 2 shows the percentage of patients with occluded or subtotally occluded infarct-related vessels and patients with patent vessels in each treatment group. There is a 15% difference between the groups in favour of the rt-PA treatment – 70% in the rt-PA-treated group and 55% in the streptokinase-treated group (95% confidence interval, +32% to −2%; $p < 0.054$).

Infusion of rt-PA resulted in a fall of the plasma fibrinogen level to $76 \pm 29\%$ (median from 2.5 to 1.8) at 60 min and to $61 \pm 35\%$ at 90 min (median 1.3) as measured with a clotting rate assay on frozen plasma samples collected with aprotinin. The plasma fibrinogen level was below 1 g/l in 1 out of 59 patients at the start of the infusion, in 8 at 60 min (13%), and in 17 at 90 min (28%). A smaller drop in the fibrinogen level was observed when measured with sodium sulphite precipitate: to $78 \pm 28\%$ at 60 min and to $69 \pm 25\%$ at 90 min (Fig. 3).

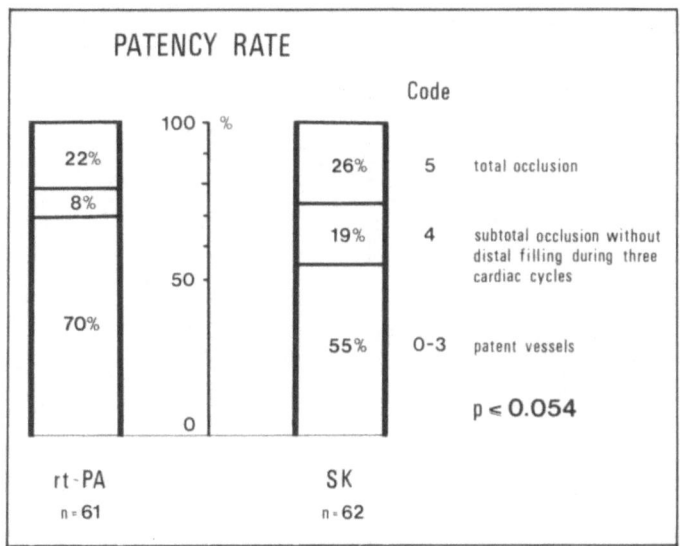

Fig. 2. Patency rate after fibrinolytic intervention. Codes 0–3 are judged as successful reperfusion

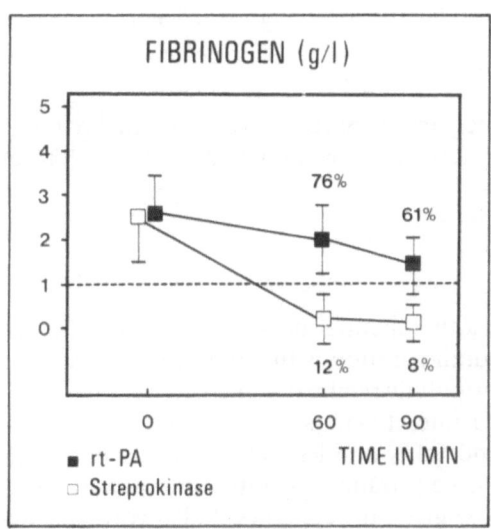

Fig. 3. Fibrinogen level at the start of the infusion and at 60 and 90 min. Comparison of rt-PA with streptokinase

Streptokinase infusion resulted in extensive systemic fibrinolytic activation as shown by a fall in fibrinogen to $12 \pm 18\%$ (median from 2.4 to 0.15) after 60 min and to $8 \pm 11\%$ after 90 min (median 0.08), with a corresponding increase of serum fibrinogen degradation products representing up to 30% of the preinfusion value of fibrinogen. With the precipitation method the fibrinogen level was $20 \pm 11\%$ of the starting value at the end of the infusion. In the streptokinase-treated group fibrinogen fell below 0.5 g/l in 54 of 62 patients (87%) at 90 min.

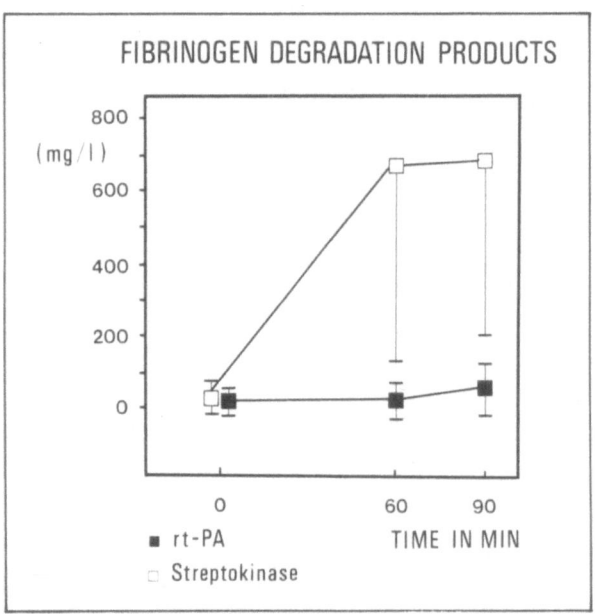

Fig. 4. Level of fibrinogen degradation products at the start of the infusion and at 60 and 90 min. Comparison of rt-PA with streptokinase

The level of fibrinogen degradation products in serum rose in rt-PA treated patients to $2.2 \pm 2.7\%$ of the baseline fibrinogen level after 60 min and to $4.6 \pm 5.2\%$ at 90 min (Fig. 4).

Discussion

One might say, if thrombolysis is to have a therapeutic role in acute myocardial infarction, the intravenous route of drug administration is the only realistic one, but since even quite a complex intravenous fibrinolytic regimen is likely to be much more widely practicable than an intracoronary route, it is important to discover whether the effect of intravenous fibrinolysis on mortality and left ventricular function can be about as great as that which is likely to be produced by intracoronary administration. The earlier that treatment could be given to reopen occluded coronary arteries and reverse ischaemia, the better. The main target is thrombolysis as rapid and complete as possible.

The dose regimen of rt-PA was selected on the only therapeutic experience available when this trial was planned and compared with a high dose, short-term intravenous infusion of streptokinase. The disadvantage of having no pretreatment coronary angiography is that visualisation of the coronary circulation after thrombolytic treatment does not allow us to establish definite reperfusion but only to compare patency rate between 2 treatment groups. With the very strict myocardial infarction criteria applied in this trial and the short duration of clinical symptoms it is likely that 80% or more of the patients at admission had an occluded vessel in the infarct area. We chose to exclude vessels with poor distal flow from our definition of

188

patency because clinical experience suggests that inadequate distal flow is irrelevant to myocardial salvage.

The 2 drug regimens were well tolerated. It is not possible to analyse whether reocclusion occurred more frequently and rapidly with 1 of the 2 treatments compared in this trial since the end-point was set at the coronary angiography obtained 90 min after the start of thrombolytic treatment and further treatment was left to the discretion of the investigator. The slightly higher incidence of arrhythmia and atrioventricular block in the rt-PA treated patients may be related to a higher reperfusion rate. The early bolus of 5.000 IU of heparin together with mechanical trauma may have caused the bleeding, which occurred mainly at the arterial puncture site. There were appreciably fewer bleeding events in the rt-PA group.

As expected, streptokinase treatment induced an intense activation of the circulating fibrinolytic system with a circulating fibrinogen level of 12% (clotting rate assay) or 20% (precipitation method) of the starting value at the end of the infusion. With 0.75 mg rt-PA/kg body weight the circulating fibrinogen at the end of the infusion fell to 61% (clotting rate assay) or 69% (precipitation method) of the value before infusion.

A remarkable discrepancy was observed between the extent of fibrinogen degradation and the appearance of degradation products. A fall in fibrinogen of 29% at 90 min in the rt-PA group corresponded to a recovery of only 4.5% as degradation products, whereas a fall in fibrinogen of 88% in the streptokinase group was associated with 30% recovery as coagulable fibrinogen degradation products. This finding suggests that fibrinogen breakdown during rt-PA infusion is less extensive, yielding molecules which are not measured in the fibrinogen assays but are nevertheless incorporated in the clot when serum is obtained for the assay of fibrinogen degradation products.

In this trial treatment with rt-PA was associated with a higher patency rate of the infarct-related vessel; the confidence interval of the difference does not exclude the possibility that rt-PA and streptokinase are in fact of equal efficacy but rt-PA treatment produced considerably less systemic fibrinolysis.

References

1. Schroeder R, Biamino G, Leitner ER et al (1983) Intravenous short-term infusion of streptokinase in acute myocardial infarction. Circulation 67:536–548
2. Verstraete M, Bernard R, Bory M et al (1985) Randomised trial of intravenous recombinant tissue-type plasminogen activator versus intravenous streptokinase in acute myocardial infarction. Lancet i:842–847

Author's address:
Prof. Dr. med. W. Rutsch
Klinikum Charlottenburg of the Freie Universitaet Berlin
Department of Cardiology
Spandauer Damm 130
1000 Berlin 19
West Germany

Panel Discussion

Chairmen: E. R. Passamani and M. Verstraete

Summary

In the first part of the panel discussion European and American studies dealing with tissue plasminogen activator (t-PA) are outlined.

It is mentioned that the main goal of the European t-PA studies was to obtain exact information on the optimal dose and the best time course of administration. In these studies (second phase) the patients received 40 mg of t-PA over 60 min. If the vessel was sufficiently patent at the time of angiography (immediately after t-PA infusion) the patients were randomly allocated to further t-PA or heparin treatment. The result was controlled by 2 further angiograms, 8–24 h after the first investigation and prior to discharge from hospital.

At present studies are being planned in Europe and in the U.S.A. dealing with more detailed questions (e.g. left ventricular function, preservation of viable myocardium).

Very important studies will investigate the value of combined t-PA and PTCA treatment in the near future.

Comparative aspects of streptokinase/urokinase and t-PA therapy were discussed. Although streptokinase and urokinase appear to be clot-sensitive reperfusion rates are low: approximately 40–50%. It is supposed that low perfusion rates will chiefly be found in patients with previous infarction and reinfarction in the same area. Despite this fact it is generally accepted that thrombolytic therapy should still be performed in individuals with previous infarction, especially if a new area of myocardium is at risk.

It is stressed that thrombolytic therapy should be initiated as early as possible.

The European Cooperative Study Group is undertaking a study of the value of t-PA in the treatment of pulmonary embolism.

DE BONO:

European t-PA studies

The rationale behind the second phase of the European t-PA studies – if you regard the placebo and streptokinase studies as parts A and B of the first phase – is really motivated by two concepts. First, we were still uncertain of how much rt-PA to give as it is an expensive drug and, secondly, we were concerned about the optimum time course of giving the drug. There is quite a lot of evidence in the literature, going back some 4 or 5 years, that serial angiography in patients who receive continuing thrombolytic treatment with, for example, streptokinase, reveals a progressive change in the nature of what was previously, for several hours, a coronary occlusion. Our rather arbitrary choice of a time point of 90 min to perform an angiogram in the first phase of the European study was based on

190

Reperfusion	our concern that there was adequate reperfusion within the time-scale which we thought would be necessary to preserve myocardium. However, this still leaves us with what in many cases looks like a fairly severe coronary stenosis, and we were anxious to see whether this could be further treated with a second infusion of t-PA.

our concern that there was adequate reperfusion within the time-scale which we thought would be necessary to preserve myocardium. However, this still leaves us with what in many cases looks like a fairly severe coronary stenosis, and we were anxious to see whether this could be further treated with a second infusion of t-PA.

Dose regimen The protocol for the second-phase trial was thus to give each patients 40 mg of t-PA over 60 min followed by an angiogram, and then, if the vessel was occluded, the patient left the study and went on to i.c. streptokinase with or without angioplasty. If the vessel was adequately patent, they were then randomized to receive either a further infusion of t-PA or heparin. A repeat angiogram was performed 8 to 24 h later with a further angiogram at the time of discharge from hospital. We have been analyzing infarct-related stenoses with a computerized stenosis analysis system in Rotterdam. The analysis of residual stenosis can be difficult after partial thrombolysis because quite often one sees thrombus in the lumen, and appropriate contours around the thrombus are not easily obtained. Since we have not yet completed the collection of data I cannot yet say whether or not the second infusion cleans up the coronary artery.

VERSTRAETE:

Left ventricular function study One of our future cooperative trials is a left ventricular function study. Two trials are being performed simultaneously, one of which is more aggressive than the other, in different centres. What are the mechanics of the simpler of these two trials?

VAN DE WERF:

t-PA vs. conventional treatment In a double-blind randomized study we intend to compare conventional coronary care unit treatment with conventional treatment supplemented by an intravenous infusion of t-PA. Both groups will receive heparin, eventually followed by coumarin. There will be no catheterization in the acute stage, but between days 10 and 21 after the experimental infusion, all patients will receive coronary angiography, left-ventricular angiography, radionuclide angiography, and an exercise test. There will be a follow-up of about one year, and we will look at reinfarction rate, PTCA, coronary bypass surgery, and of course mortality. This is thus a simple protocol with no catheterization in the acute stage.

VERSTRAETE:

In principle, we would have 200 patients in each arm. We now turn to the more aggressive trial.

SIMOONS:

**t-PA
and
PTCA**

It is clear that thrombolysis opens vessels but we are not yet sure about the total cost-benefit relation because of certain additional costs in the follow-up of patients. If we could show that thrombo-lytic therapy with t-PA is superior to placebo, the next question should be if it is necessary to add PTCA to the treatment. In order to study this question properly we would like to do a study with some 10 or 12 centres which have great experience and skill in PTCA, and to compare patients treated with intravenous t-PA only, with patients treated with intravenous t-PA rapidly followed within 1 or 2 h by angiography and PTCA. PTCA might then fur-ther increase the number of patent vessels and would certainly in-

**Infarct
size**

crease the degree of patency. The formal major endpoints in both studies will be function and estimated infarct size, while the other clinical data will be considered as an additional endpoint. The stud-ies will probably not be large enough to show an effect on survival, but they certainly will be large enough to show any effect on global and left ventricular function and to estimate the effect on infarct size.

VERSTRAETE:

**Data Centre
Rotterdam**

Dr. Lubsen assembles all study data at the Data Centre in Rotter-dam. How is this done?

LUBSEN:

**European
Cooperative
Study
Group**

To start with the background of the European Cooperative Study Group and how it was initiated, the basic idea behind the group was to achieve some uniformity of definition between the various stud-ies. It was not at all our intention to set up a large clinical trial bu-reaucracy that everybody has to follow. In addition, the idea was to assemble in one place certain types of core data that would enable us to follow all known applications of the drug for a number of years to come to study certain rates of disease, especially known cor-onary disease, that may be very important in the future. The prob-lem with this type of study is that the people who decide upon the protocol do not perform it in practice. It is necessary to set up a sys-tem to ensure flawless execution of the protocol, which we have achieved by avoiding the usual pile of forms and manuals of oper-ation, and instead writing out a very specific, detailed list of step by step instructions. Besides a space in which the data are to be re-corded, there are also general procedural instructions as to what to do if side-effects develop and so on. This system has worked very well. For the studies we have just discussed we will simply continue it and modify it as necessary but the general principle will stay the same. In addition, as before, we will use "blinded" assessment of all primary endpoint related films and data in the Zurich Centre. All the assessments of the endpoints will be done centrally and independently by people not working in the clinics.

PASSAMANI:

I must say the Europeans certainly have given us plenty of stimulation in the last two years. First as Dr. Verstraete said, by developing this new elixir, and secondly by settling, it seems, the question about thrombolytic therapy, at least acutely.

HEROOK:

TIMI
phase II

Dr. Passamani, you said that phase II of the TIMI study would be testing the benefit of thrombolysis on the quantity and quality of life. Is this to be tested against a placebo or heparin? Or do you intend to test two thrombolytic agents?

PASSAMANI:

Based on discussions with our investigative group, and having heard the results of GISSI, we have reluctantly concluded that it would be very difficult to perform a placebo controlled trial in America today. It will be even more difficult six months from now when GISSI is available to everyone. We are therefore moving, as the European group is, towards a design which can overcome what I call the "morning after" problem. When we treat a patient with thrombolytic therapy, have we treated one disease and caused another? That is, is the patient going to go home for his second, or recurrent infarction when that artery closes down? We are progres-

t-PA
and PTCA

sing towards a trial in which all patients will receive t-PA, with a decision to randomize to PTCA or not, and will probably look at long-term survival free of recurrent infarction. The design issue is very difficult.

HEROOK:

Dr. Van de Werf, do you intend to use placebo?

VAN DE WERF:

It will be a placebo control with randomized study, yes.

PASSAMANI:

Again, I must emphasize that it is with sadness that we abandoned placebo use. We were very concerned that if we tried to push a placebo controlled trial into the current ambience in America we would end up with a highly selected group of patients: high risk, early anterior MIs would be bled away from the trial, and we would end up in the very difficult position of not knowing to which population our results could be applied.

ERBEL:

Low reperfusion rate after streptokinase

Dr. Passamani, the low reperfusion rate with streptokinase is astonishing. Is this fact related to the high percentage of patients with previous myocardial infarction in your group? The number reached nearly 20%. And what is the reperfusion rate if you exclude these patients?

PASSAMANI:

We were also very surprised by that reperfusion rate. I asked our statisticians to do a sample size calculation based on two assumptions. One is one-third reduction by giving thrombolytic therapy on in-hospital mortality; the second assumption is that only 40 or 50% of the arteries given streptokinase will open. This produces a 20% reduction, which is what the Italian group saw. Also, it should be emphasized that TIMI is a late trial, with a mean time of delivery of four and three quarter hours. In contrast most of the Italian trial related to early treated patients. There may be a difference there.

VON ESSEN:

Early administration of streptokinase

From our experience we know that streptokinase given within the first one or two hours obviously has a higher reperfusion rate than if you give it later on. In your special trial you have an occlusion time of more than four hours. Do you think that this is one of the reasons why your reperfusion rate with streptokinase is not very high?

PASSAMANI:

The answer ist that in TIMI, streptokinase given at an average of four and three quarter hours is not a very good thrombolytic agent. The question of whether we could have given it earlier and obtained a better result cannot be answered, since we have very small numbers of patients treated earlier. We have 10% treated in less than three hours, 35% in less than four hours.

GÖRKER:

Different infusion times of t-PA and streptokinase

The duration of the infusion of t-PA and streptokinase differed in the TIMI trial and the European trial, with only a 60 min streptokinase infusion versus a 90 min t-PA infusion. That means the infusion was done for 30 min before the angiogram was taken and there is a possibility of reocclusion during this time period. What is your opinion of this?

DE BONO:

**t-PA and
heparin**

**t-PA
and
streptokinase**

When we started planning these trials, because of variable data and
a lack of personnel experienced in giving t-PA, we went through a
variety of different dose schedules. The administration of t-PA was
followed by an infusion of heparin. This is tremendously important
because although, of course, streptokinase gives an on-going anticoagulant effect, the anticoagulant effect of t-PA stops very shortly
after the infusion is stopped. The question of the length of the infusion and the effects of its length on the degree of resolution of the
obstruction is something that the second phase trial is looking at
very specifically. When we chose the streptokinase dose and duration we really took en bloc what at that stage seemed to be the best
conventional streptokinase administration policy, the Schroeder
protocol.

PASSAMANI:

When we designed our trial, 1.5 million units given over an hour was
the dose that both hematologists and experienced cardiologists recommended. This dose was also used in the Italien study.

GANZ:

**Reopening
rates**

I hope that t-PA will be better than streptokinase, but I still think
that for clarification, there is a distortion caused by time. It is clear
that urokinase and streptokinase are much more clot sensitive than
t-PA, and that streptokinase applied early and followed for a long
time can obtain a reopening rate in excess of 90%. I would expect
that t-PA, when applied properly, will attain the same rate. However, the thrombolytic process is very complex and detailed. When
these studies are designed, details are not always carefully prepared.
Such details include anticoagulation. Not enough attention is paid
to reocclusion. I think that when we start the new trial we should
pay more attention to these details, or they may destroy the major
impact of the procedure itself.

VERSTRAETE:

**Side-
effects**

There are two points I think I should clarify here. First, in our
group, at least, we have no evidence that scu-PA or pro-urokinase
is more fibrin specific than t-PA. In our animal experiments it is
slightly less fibrin specific. Secondly, before we make any recom-
mendation for a more general use of even a more fibrin specific
thrombolytic agent, we should have more insight into possible side-
effects of these agents in clinical situations where there is no myo-

195

cardial infarction, but a ruptured aneurysm; for instance, acute pancreatitis, acute pneumonia in elderly people. How safe would t-PA, pro-urokinase and the newcomers be in these situations? Hopefully there will be no major disasters, but we cannot guarantee this.

PASSAMANI:

I think that Dr. Ganz's point about details is very important, and when we are designing a study we pay a great deal of attention to them. TIMI had a lot of bleeding, and although part of that may have been a learning curve, part of it may be accurate reporting. Side-effects, particularly bad side-effects, are something that physicians find hard to report. TIMI is realistic. We may have overestimated the amount of bleeding at the groin because we reported every instance, some of them very minor. But our group spent an enormous amount of time trying to get the details down properly so that we would not be causing patients undue difficulty.

LEVIN:

Follow-up treatment

In the TIMI trial you changed from heparin to anti-platelet drugs: was there any problem of reinfarction during this time of changing? And for how may days did you give heparin? Did you have discussions about whether anticoagulation with coumarin may have been better? And what did the GISSI group use?

PASSAMANI:

In TIMI, heparin was given until hospital discharge catheterization, and then an immediate switchover to aspirin and dipyridamole was made.

ROVELLI:

GISSI

In the GISSI trial only a few centres gave heparin and anticoagulant therapy after the treatment with streptokinase. We intend to analyse these data, but analysis or follow-up at 6 and 12 months are most important.

SIMOONS:

Dr. Rovelli, there were to differences between your data and ours. You did not have a beneficial effect in reinfarctions, and you did not have an effect in patients with an inferior wall infarct, while in both groups in our study there was an effect on mortality and on functional infarct size.

196

ROVELLI:

As concerns the incidence of reinfarction, we have seen that its incidence is greater in treated groups. In many patients treated with streptokinase, if the subsequent heparin dosage was not correct, it resulted in infarction. As to the location of the infarction, I cannot explain the low effect in inferior infarction.

Question:

Dr. Mauri, regarding the group of patients with previous infarctions, which is always very large, you did not have any effect on survival, is that correct?

MAURI:

We have had no effect on previous infarction but it is a small group in comparison to many others.

PASSAMANI:

TIMI

Our study was not designed to test the question just in patients with prior infarction. When dealing with subgroups you must be very careful.

LUBSEN:

Subgroup analysis

Subgroup analysis cannot be avoided, for two reasons. First of all you may have a study that is negative in the overall sense because there is a positive subgroup and a negative subgroup in terms of effect, and that may be a very credible effect which we can explain by everything we know about the epidemiology of the disease. The second reason that this is unavoidable is that you want to apply these results to real patients.

PASSAMANI:

Perhaps another question is whether the incidence of thrombosis in that particular group of patients is different compared to first infarcts.

HUGENHOLTZ:

Thrombolytic therapy in patients with previous infarctions?

The information that a previous infarct has taken place is, in a clinical sense, often rather easy to obtain. If, as supported by the Dutch trial, groups with previous infarcts do not do very well, and if it is true that sooner or later we have to start planning something in terms of practical recommendations, would the panel perhaps say

197

if they agree that patients who have had a previous infarct should not be given thrombolytic therapy, on the basis of current evidence?

SIMOONS:

Perhaps I should be more specific about what we did with previous infarcts in the trial in the Netherlands. About 20% of the patients had previous infarcts. These were predominantly patients with previous infarct in another area than the present infarct, and I think we should be careful to make that distinction. It is likely that if there is already a major transmural anterior wall infarct, and the patient reinfarcts in the same area, then the benefits of thrombolytic therapy might be rather small, unless there are means, and the time, to distinguish between the previously damaged myocardium and the new myocardium which is at risk or is ischemic. On the other hand, a patient with previous inferior wall infarct, and now an anterior infarct, will certainly benefit as much or probably more than a patient with a first infarct in the anterior region.

PASSAMANI:

Implicit in Dr. Hugenholtz's question is that thrombolytic therapy is going to be given to patients with acute infarction, that is, the question has now changed; instead of being why, it is now why not?

UEBIS:

Inclusion criteria

I should like to refer to the inclusion criteria and the indications for thrombolysis. In the Italian study there were quite different inclusion criteria concerning time course. Another difference to the European trials is the ECG criteria. You have very low and very small ST-segment changes as inclusion criteria, so you have to expect a rather large number of patients who have no complete thrombotic obstruction of the infarcted vessel. On the other hand this means a larger number of patients who have some kind of unstable angina. Do you have any findings differentiating the outcome of those patients, i.e. development of signs of transmural myocardial infarction, Q-waves, enzyme release and so on?

ROVELLI:

For ECG criteria we have adopted the criteria suggested by NEIH. We have verified that infarction is present. Definite infarction is verified by CPK elevation in 95% of patients, so I think that all of our patients have a definite infarction.

DE BONO:

When we first thought of doing thrombolysis we were very concerned that we should not be doing harm, particularly in hemorrhagic infarcts and so on. Perhaps we should not get too far away from that possibility simply because overall we have an improvement in survival. We recently started to use nuclear magnetic resonance to observe the myocardium following thrombolysis. We are a little concerned that in a group of patients who are treated relatively late after the onset of symptoms, we are seeing a rather worrying and persistent change in the relaxation patterns in the myocardium, which suggests that we may actually be doing harm in this subgroup. This may be particularly relevant to patients in whom there is already some loss of myocardial function because of a previous infarct. So it may well be that we should look very carefully at thrombolysis results in patients with previous infarcts to establish the relationship between the outcome and the time at which therapy is instituted.

VERSTRAETE:

t-PA and pulmonary embolism

One of the plans of the European Cooperative Study Group on t-PA is a study on pulmonary embolism. We want to try two pilot trials. One would be on life-threatening massive acute pulmonary embolism, that means those patients who are going to die under your hands. This would be an open trial of a 2 h infusion of t-PA, with then heart surgeon performing an embolectomy, if it is still necessary. The second trial would be on latent, not acute, major, not massive, pulmonary embolism. It will be more or less similar to the Ubet trial in America several years ago with streptokinase. In the massive pulmonary embolism trial t-PA will be given in the pulmonary catheter. In the other trial it will be given intravenously. These will be open trials so that we have a baseline for more formally organized comparative trials in the not too distant future. We would like to launch this trial very early in January and close it probably 4 or 6 months later.

Finally, I would like to publicly thank the members of the European Steering Committee on t-PA. These members have been extremely efficient and devoted in helping to set up and publish the trials. The reocclusion trial will be reported at the end of January, and we hope to have the pulmonary embolism trials performed and published in 1986. The left ventricle studies will probably take one and a half to two years.

What have we learned during this symposium?

1. W. Kübler

Medizinische Klinik, Ruprecht-Karls-Universität, Heidelberg (West Germany)

Many excellent studies were presented at this symposium and it is impossible to summarize them all. I will therefore concentrate on three major problems and on the solutions which have been achieved.

It has been well documented during this symposium that thrombolytic therapy may be effective in limiting infarct size and in improving prognosis, at least in a subgroup of patients.

My first point is that it is nowadays almost generally accepted that probably the most important determinant for a good functional result is early reperfusion of the infarcting area. Irreversible myocardial damage is related to depletion of high energy phosphates and accumulation of toxic products such as, for instance, lactate. Reperfusion may exaggerate the necrotic process by generation of free radicals. Enzyme systems involved may be inhibited, e.g. xanthine oxidase by allopurinol. It has been shown in animal experiments that infarct size can be limited in this way. Activation of scavenger pathways may be an alternative and perhaps additive approach. In order to reduce the reperfusion damage, thrombolysis has to be initiated early and should not only be available to patients in the large hospitals (where the studies described at this meeting were carried out) but also to patients in smaller hospitals. IV thrombolysis may be the treatment of choice, it should involve little risk, i.e. few or no systemic effects. These prerequisites may also be at least partially fulfilled by several new drugs, such as pro-urokinase, which has no apparent affinity to fibrin and is activated by catalytic amounts of plasmin in the immediate surroundings of the thrombus; t-PA, with a high affinity to fibrin which only induces plasminogen activation at the fibrin surface; or active urokinase bound to a fibrin-specific monoclonal antibody. With some of these new drugs, mainly with t-PA, clinical results were presented, and the studies performed with t-PA are at least very encouraging.

Secondly, the results obtained by thrombolytic treatment must be evaluated by different criteria. Reduction in mortality would be the most valuable, but is also the most time-consuming and the most expensive end-point. In contrast to animal experiments, limitation of infarct size is not easily proved in humans. First we have to define hemodynamic parameters. Evaluation of regional wall motion seems to be superior to the determination of global or even regional ejection fraction in order to demonstrate salvage of threatened myocardium. Exercise studies may further improve the sensitivity of the techniques. Secondly, metabolic parameters for the evaluation of coronary flow or perfusion also have to be established for the evaluation of certain metabolic activities and/or of cell necrosis using isotope cardiography. For a good spatial resolution tomographic techniques should be applied. For any marker, however, its kinetics under normal and ischemic conditions have to be elaborated. Thirdly, ECG mapping or two dimensional echocardiography may be not as sensitive as the hemodynamic or metabolic techniques. The two methods, however, are non-invasive and therefore easily applied. They are also rather cheap. In any case we have to bear in mind that activity of certain metabolic pathways, viability, and pump function are not identical functional end-points, and may not be well correlated.

Finally, if early reperfusion of the infarcting area can be initiated, reocclusion of the infarcting area may occur. Thirty-eight per cent – as mentioned during this symposium – has to be considered as an old but honest figure. Eighty per cent of these patients may have signs of reinfarction and this again indicates salvage of infarcting myocardium by early thrombolysis. As a risk of reocclusion of the residual stenosis cannot be predicted in the individual patient, general measures have to be applied. Most experience is available with PTCA. This measure bears a small risk of reocclusion in itself, but this is less than 5%. Nowadays, most studies indicate improvement of long-term results and of prognosis by early PTCA of the residual stenosis. The same applies to bypass surgery which can be performed with a hospital mortality of less than 2%. These positive trends had to be confirmed by randomized controlled trials; especially for bypass surgery after thrombolysis, however, the methodological problems for such a study can almost not be overestimated. Medical treatment to keep the vessels open and PTCA or bypass surgery are not alternative but rather additive regimes. Medical treatment may either be directed to reduce vasomotor tone and/or to reduce rethrombosis and progression of the arteriosclerotic process. The effective treatment has still to be established.

Author's address:
Prof. Dr. W. Kübler
Medizinische Klinik
Abteilung Innere Medizin III
Ruprecht-Karls-Universität
Bergheimer Straße 58
6900 Heidelberg
West Germany

What have we learned during this symposium?

2. J. Lubsen

Department of Cardiology (Thoraxcenter), Erasmus University,
Rotterdam (The Netherlands)

If this symposium had been a court trial I would be willing to defend the following statement: early thrombolysis is efficacious in patients with acute myocardial infarction because it improves left ventricular function, reduces the incidence of complications and reduces mortality. Later on, I will modify this statement when I come to the question of practical recommendations. But for the moment this is the statement I am going to defend. As is usual in court, a distinction is made between key evidence on the one hand and corroborating evidence on the other. As far as key evidence is concerned, two studies must be mentioned. These are, in random order, the Italian GISSI trial and the trial by the Interuniversity Cardiology Institute in the Netherlands. On their own these two studies would perhaps not offer sufficient key evidence, but taken together they fit a pattern. What is most important in this pattern is this: the earlier thrombolysis is started, the greater the effect, which is in agreement with clinical experience and results from animal experiments. Many of the other studies that we have heard about these days I would list as corroborating evidence. In particular, one would point at the relationship between opening up coronary arteries in acute myocardial infarction on the one hand and improved left ventricular function and prognosis on the other as corroborating evidence. With all these results taken together, I think any court would agree that the case at hand is rather strong.

Certainly, we have heard about problems too. One of the most important problems that needs to be resolved seems to be the question of reperfusion damage. Some papers have been presented about the possible mechanisms. It is important to stress that animal experiments have shown that myocardial preservation can only be achieved when recanalization is applied quickly after onset; with increasing occlusion time, less myocardium is saved and there is a possibility that after a certain point in time, recanalization even increases infarct size. It is perhaps not unreasonable to assume that reperfusion damage per se is not related to the type of thrombolytic agent used. A second problem which is definitely related to the agent is the incidence of side effects. Streptokinase seems to be worse in this regard than some of the newer agents, in particular tissue-type plasminogen activator, but the real benefits of the latter remain to be established. A third problem is the efficacy of thrombolytic agents when they are used intravenously. For eventual widespread application, a thrombolytic agent is needed that is effective when used in this way. As far as this aspect is concerned, there is now convincing evidence that in particular tissue-type plasminogen activator is much better than streptokinase. A fourth problem that should be mentioned here is the risk of rethrombosis. Most likely, this risk is not only related to the degree of residual stenosis, but also to the agent that was used and the concomitant management as far as anticoagulation is concerned. Much further work seems to be needed to clarify exactly what determines rethrombosis and how it can be prevented. It is noted in this context that this is not a new problem. It is the old problem of secondary prevention in a new disguise.

During this symposium the thrombolytic agents that are now available were extensively discussed. Most people would agree that tissue-type plasminogen activator is at the moment the most promising. I have mentioned already that it seems to be more effective after intravenous administration than streptokinase. Some have argued that the risk of side effects such as bleeding is not really reduced after the application of tissue-type plasminogen activator. I think that it is rather too early to be conclusive as far as this is concerned. So far, tissue-type plasminogen activator has only been used in extensively instrumented patients who received full anticoagulation in addition to TPA. The real picture as far as bleeding risk is concerned will only emerge when tissue-type plasminogen activator is used in controlled studies which do not employ acute catheterization.

What then should be the message to the practitioner that comes out of this meeting? We can tell the practising physicians in the field that as far as one issue is concerned there seems to be general agreement: both intravenous and intracoronary thrombolysis is efficacious and can be used in medical practice, provided that the use is limited to early administration in patients with typical infarcts. But we should be very careful in promoting this indication. At present, there is no evidence that there is still a positive effect when thrombolysis is started after, say, 6 h. In addition thrombolysis has not been studied in patients who have less clear-cut signs of infarction than the ones spelled out in the inclusion criteria of the studies reported so far. Furthermore, it is open to question whether, for instance, inferior infarcts really benefit. But if one heeds these precautions, thrombolysis can now be recommended. The second thing that we should tell the practitioners is that there is also controversy. At this meeting, the view was heard that thrombolysis can only be effective if it is followed immediately by acute catheterization and PTCA. Admittedly, some clinics have very good experience with this procedure. On the other hand, it has to be realized that if this view point is really correct, the scope of application of thrombolysis will be limited not by the number of patients who sustain myocardial infarction, but by the availability of facilities to do these procedures within the short time-span that is available. It seems likely that this controversy will be resolved in the near future. Trials are being planned or are under way which compare thrombolysis plus early PTCA with thrombolysis alone.

Author's address:
Professor J. Lubsen, M.D.
Thoraxcenter Bd 381
Clinical Epidemiology Unit
Erasmus Universiteit Rotterdam
Postbus 1738
3000 DR Rotterdam
The Netherlands

What shall we recommend to the practising physician and the cardiologist in a general hospital?

1. D. G. Julian

Freeman Hospital, Newcastle-Upon-Tyne (United Kingdom)

I have been asked to address the question of what we should tell the physicians in practice today, bearing in mind the facilities and drugs which are presently available. This excludes rt-PA and any of the newer strategies. As I see it, we have four options. First, we can tell physicians to do nothing. Secondly, we can advise them to use intravenous streptokinase. Thirdly, we can suggest they use intracoronary streptokinase or fourthly we can suggest intracoronary or intravenous streptokinase plus PTCA.

Sir Winston Churchill said that the oldest habit in the world for resisting change is to complain that unless the remedy can be universally applied it should not be applied at all. I think this is highly appropriate to the discussions in this publication. Although it might be said that intracoronary streptokinase is an impractical form of therapy, many coronary care units have portable image intensifiers of sufficient quality for it to be possible to perform intracoronary injections and intracoronary thrombolysis. Indeed, in a number of places, for instance in Glasgow, this is actually used. So it is not an impossible form of therapy and if it is the best, then we should use it where it is available, even if it is not universally available.

The Western Washington Trial has been splendidly devised and carried out but the 1 year mortality rates (i.c. streptokinase group: 8.2%, control group: 14.7%, $p = 0.17$, n.s.) show that there was not a significant benefit from this form of therapy at that time. It is true that if one looks at subsets defined retrospectively one can see benefits in certain subgroups. But what to my mind is more worrying is that there is a significant randomisation problem: significantly more people were randomised to streptokinase. Furthermore, the control group was unnecessarily submitted to coronary arteriography in the acute phase. I do not feel, therefore, that we can determine from this, whether we should be using intracoronary streptokinase or not.

In the Dutch study, death had occurred in 10% of patients on conventional therapy by 14 days. By contrast, only 5% of 'thrombolysis' patients had died by 14 days, a significant result. Unfortunately, however, the problem is a little more complicated than that. A peculiar feature of this trial is that ventricular fibrillation occurred in 23 per cent of the control group. Since seeing the results of this trial, I have investigated our own material, looking at a similar time slot and using similar ECG criteria. Our incidence is 8 per cent, even though we do not use lidocain, so this figure of 23 per cent is very high. Before we accept these data as a baseline for our actions we should ask the Dutch study group to explain why their patients fibrillated so often. In terms of mortality there is no question that this study is very impressive. However, the trial was a complex one with many variables, the treated group receiving several forms of therapy, apart from streptokinase, that the control group did not. The treated group did better than the control group but it is not possible to conclude from this trial that it was streptokinase per se that was responsible.

Another criterion by which we judge intravenous streptokinase is left ventricular function. I view measurements of left ventricular function as a useful procedure. They should reflect the patient's ability to be free of left ventricular symptoms which require surgery or PTCA, or which lead to reinfarction. In the Dutch study a total of 102 patients had PTCA or bypass surgery. In fact, non fatal reinfarction is also very much higher in the thrombolysis group (36, versus 16 in the control group). So when we say we are improving left ventricular function, one is using the term left ventricular function in a rather special sense. I consider that at the moment there is no good case for recommending the widespread use of intracoronary streptokinase, even where it is available. On the other hand, there is quite a good case for those centres which are capable of using the complete Dutch package to do so. I would therefore agree with von Essen's view, that if one is going to go ahead with coronary angiography, one should also go ahead with PTCA or whatever seems appropriate.

In the Yusuf review (2) all the studies with intracoronary streptokinase are examined, apart from the latest data from the Dutch study. There was no significant benefit from intracoronary streptokinase (a pooled result of 12.5% mortality in the treated patients compared to 14.7% in controls) whereas even before GISSI (1) the data favoured a benefit from intravenous streptokinase (a pooled mortality rate of 15.4% in treated patients versus 19.2% in controls). Now that we have GISSI, I think we feel more confident that we are achieving something very real with intravenous streptokinase.

The question arises here as to how we translate clinical trials into clinical practice. One of the problems of course is that clinical trials never prove anything, they only supply probabilities. Furthermore, in applying clinical trials to practice, one is obliged to use extrapolation, which is not an exact science. In my view we now have enough information, and a sufficiently good theoretical basis to recommend the use of i.v. streptokinase to physicians who do not have intracoronary streptokinase or at least PTCA available to them. This treatment can be particularly recommended for use in those groups for which GISSI and other studies suggest it is of most value. With regard to time delay, I feel that under 4 hours is appropriate, but clearly, our most important task is to reorganize our health services to bring patients to hospital more quickly, so that we can give intravenous streptokinase to those who are most likely to benefit.

References

1. Gruppo Italiano per lo Studio della Streptochinasi nell' Infarcto Miocardio (GISSI) (1986) Effectiveness of intravenous thrombolytic treatment in acute myocardial infarction. Lancet i:397–402
2. Yusuf S, Collins R, Peto R et al (1985) Intravenous and intracoronary fibrinolytic therapy in acute myocardial infarction: overview of results on mortality, re-infarction and side-effects from 33 randomized controlled trials. Eur Heart J 6:556–583

Author's address:
Professor D. G. Julian
Department of Cardiology
Freeman Hospital
Freeman Road
High Heaton
Newcastle upon Tyne, NE7 7DN
United Kingdom

What shall we recommend to the practising physician and the cardiologist in a general hospital?

2. P. G. Hugenholtz

Akademisch Ziekenhuis, Thoraxcentrum, Rotterdam (The Netherlands)

The doctor working in the general hospital, not necessarily the doctor out in practice in the smaller towns, sees a great deal of patients and has a very difficult decision to make in the use of thrombolysis in acute myocardial infarction. He may feel bewildered, sometimes bemused, and certainly at times very confused. Dr Sonnenblick has said that he feels that the credibility of the medical profession is threatened by our conflicting reflections of what we investigate and what we find. It is, in my view, an unavoidable situation because what we are seeing is the mixing of research information on the experimental animal level with the signals coming from humans. No experimental animal can ever mimic the human situation (and the comments about collateral flow being important are absolutely correct), as long ago pointed out by Kübler. The data we obtain from the better designed trials, not perhaps the best, are still informative because they provide us with an insight, even though they are often conflicting. Now we have the culmination of the work in randomised trials which could give us, perhaps, the final answer. However, so often these trials seem to have a population that is no longer recognizable, at least in some of the better designed trials, I did not recognize my patients. I do not see control mortalities of 4 percent for myocardial infarction occurring in a general hospital. That might not mean that they do not exist, but it is not difficult to understand how the community at large feels that we are giving inconsistent signals. The most reliable and expensive trials do not relate to the problem that we in practice see. So what do we do in practice? The first thing to realize is that at present a straight answer is unobtainable, because opinions are still changing and changing very rapidly. Secondly, I personally would feel pushed from behind by my colleagues who say: "No, don't do something when you don't think it is a good idea." On the other hand they ask if something new is not available, and this is a continuous force that pushes forward. We as specialists in that regional hospital must decide upon a course. So option number one, wait, see, and stay with conventional therapy is out. And I agree fully with Professor Julian that, at this particular point, we should move, so if I were in a peripheral hospital, I would be supported by two major pieces of evidence that I heard at this conference. I am convinced from the GISSI and the Dutch data that a strategy aimed at early reperfusion is by now incontrovertibly a beneficial procedure. So I have to go in that direction and prepare my community accordingly.

The evidence we had in the Dutch trial, namely the decrease of ventricular fibrillation rate, but also more importantly, the decreased incidence of cardiac failure and the halving of cardiogenic shock, have changed morbidity in a significant sense. This gives me personally the greatest urge to move on in this direction, because in addition to saving lives, the community, the authorities, and the patient can be saved a lot of problems. If we stay with a calculation like Dr. Klein's, we are too limited. He was incomplete because he failed to acknowledge that many of these units already exist and they are often not doing anything at the hours we might need to use them. We should put our house in order much more effectively, the plea Desmond Julian made, since we already have the physical resources.

Secondly, we can save in terms of avoiding unnecessary complications. Why wait to treat somebody in shock with a balloon pump etc. when you know that he has a 50 percent chance of dying in one year and that it costs 40 000 $ just to keep him alive for the first six months. And that is a conservative estimate. So I think the second argument for me to go along with the reperfusion strategy would be that I know that I would reduce the morbidity and the complication rate, as well as ultimately saving money.

The third step would mean talking to my collegues in the community. I have to talk to my transportation system, I have to talk to the general public. I have to initiate a total systems re-think. These are common terms in the business and technical world, but not for doctors in the medical world. They really do not think in these terms. We seem to be a haphazard collection of items and individuals, which could be far better structured. If we had done this some time ago I think we could all get these rapid arrival times that we have shown to be the greatest benefit of all.

I would then, if I had that system more or less organized, go and treat my patients. But I would reserve my initial attempt as a general physician in a general hospital to the patients with whom I would be most likely to succeed. I would refuse to lyse, although it sounds a bit radical, those who arrived too late. I would try to get the patients into the hospital before the fourth hour. I would limit myself initially to the anterior large infarctions, not only because they show the greatest benefit but also because that is the group where the whole subsequent PTCA procedure or surgery seems to have the greatest efficacy. So the whole system will be benefiting from that as well. I would begin by limiting myself to the younger age groups and I should absolutely insist on having a referral system to a catheterization laboratory so that if the i.v. streptokinase or t-PA was given previously, perhaps by the GP or in the ambulance, and the patient came to my hospital, I would know what to do. When he or she did *not* belong to the 60 percent who indeed lysed and then cooled off, but remained hot, and had pain again, then they should be able to go to angiography and/or PTCA or surgery. And I would want to have that chance behind me, to be supported in the rear. If I did not have that, I probably would *not* carry out the above procedures.

So, to sum up, I would like to change certain things in my community, so that I could employ the best lessons presented at this conference. But I am forced to admit that, whether I like it or not, I must progress. I must move to a strategy of early reperfusion and I must try to implement it optimally in the focus of the setting as I find it.

Author's address:
Professor P. G. Hugenholtz
Akademisch Ziekenhuis
Thoraxcentrum
Molewaterplein 40
3015 DG Rotterdam
The Netherlands

What should the health services and regulatory agencies take into account?

H. H. Klein and H. Kreuzer

Klinikum der Universität Göttingen (West Germany)

It is generally accepted that in most patients with acute myocardial infarction only reperfusion therapy offers the chance to reduce myocardial infarct size and mortality. Before we begin to calculate the costs of different thrombolytic treatments, we must try to outline the possible beneficial effect of reperfusion on infarct size. If the results of collateral or residual blood flow at the acute event are superimposed on the development of infarcts in different animal species with a known amount of collateral blood flow, we can expect the following pattern of infarct development (2).
Figure 1 shows that three groups of patients can be separated. Group A has no angiographically visible collateral blood flow, group B has a faint visible collateral blood flow, and group C has good collateral or residual blood flow. About 40% of the patients with acute myocardial infarction belong to group A, 35% to group B, and the remaining 25% to group C. Ultimate infarct size in group A is supposed to be reached within 90 min of ischemia, and is about 85–100% when considered as the percentage of the risk region. In group B, final infarct size will be reached within 3 hours and is in the range of 60–85%. Ultimate infarct size in group C varies between 0 or 1% and 60%. In group C it is difficult or impossible to predict when the final infarct size is reached. Figure 1 suggests that reperfusion after 90 min of ischemia may reduce infarct size in about 60% of the patients, and reperfusion after 3 h of ischemia reduces infarct size in only 25% of the patients. The benefits of early treat-

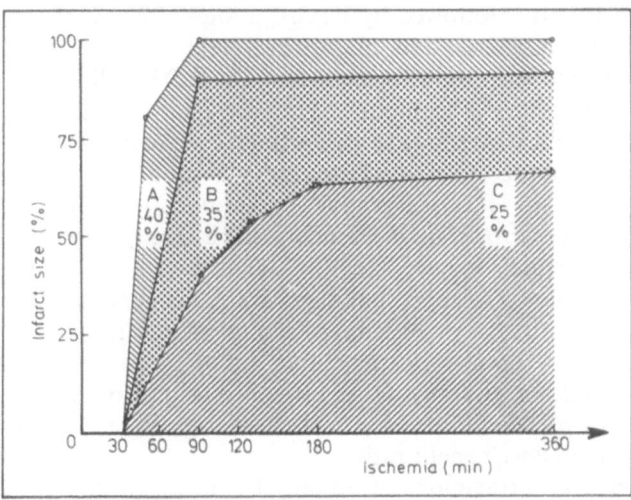

Fig. 1. Separation of three groups of patients according to collateral or residual blood flow. Reproduced from Klein, H.H., Kreuzer, H. (1986). Deutsch Med Wschr. 111:270–272, with kind permission from Georg Thieme Verlag, Stuttgart (2).

ment (a reduction in mortality by about 20% and a reduction in congestive heart failure by about 50%) are clearly demonstrated by the GISSI and Dutch trials. The analysis of the relationship between costs and benefits of different reperfusion strategies is rendered difficult by the fact that there are no randomized trials comparing these treatments in relation to infarct size or mortality. That means that a comparison has not been made between systemic and intracoronary thrombolysis, or between systemic and systemic/intracoronary thrombolysis with or without acute PTCA. Therefore we can only summarize the costs of different strategies (Table 1).

Table 1. Costs of i.v. thrombolytic therapy

1) Medicaments	a) Streptokinase	1,5 Mill U	258 DM (purchase price)
	Cortisol	500 mg	25 DM (purchase price)
	b) Urokinase	2 Mill U	1085 DM (purchase price)
2) Staff	No additonal personnel required		

Intravenous thrombolytic therapy represents by far the cheapest approach, especially because no additional personnel is required. The cost of tissue-plasminogen activator is not known because it is not yet for sale, but we can expect that it will be quite expensive.

The costs increase dramatically if intracoronary treatment is offered 24 hours per day. The employer pays about 95 000 DM a year for the staff on call, consisting of two doctors, one nurse, and one technical assistant. If all of the eighty catheterization laboratories in West Germany (1) had members of staff on call, the cost would be 7.5 million DM per year. The average calculated costs for one intracoronary thrombolysis is about 4000 DM. If it is followed by PTCA, another 2000 DM has to be added. If each of the eighty catheterization laboratories treat 50 patients per year (i.e. a total of 4000 patients per year) the enormous amount of 23 million DM has to be taken into account. Alongside the high costs of intracoronary thrombolysis, it must be noted that only a small percentage of patients with acute myocardial infarction can be treated by this method, if we accept the time limit of about 3–4 h between the onset of symptoms and the start of therapy. Furthermore, each department must have 4 to 6 experienced doctors available, rendering this therapy very impracticable. We conclude the following:

Ischemic tolerance of the myocardium is so short that in general, only very early reperfusion, e.g. within 2 or 2 to 4 hours, salvages jeopardized myocardium. Even a covering network of catheterization laboratories available for every patient at a maximum distance of 25 km could not guarantee that intracoronary thrombolysis could be started early enough to reduce infarct size in the majority of cases. This treatment is characterized by a high cost/benefit ratio.

Reperfusion frequency is lower with intravenous thrombolysis. However, this therapy can be started earlier and is relatively inexpensive. Combined i.v.-i.c. thrombolysis is a promising approach. At present cost/benefit estimations, especially in comparison to intravenous thrombolysis with newer agents, would be premature.

212

References

1. Dörr R, Effert S, v Essen R, Ahnert F, Tolxdorff T (1985) Intrakoronare thrombolytische Therapie des akuten Myokardinfarktes. Deutsch Ärzteblatt 41:2329–2334
2. Klein HH, Kreuzer H (1986) Neue Aspekte zum zeitlichen Verlauf der Myokardinfarktentwicklung. Deutsch Med Wschr 111:270–272

Author's address:

H. H. Klein, M.D.
Med. Klinik und Poliklinik
Klinikum der Universität Göttingen
Robert-Koch-Straße 40
3400 Göttingen
West Germany

Discussion

MESSMER:

About 15 to 20 years ago it was said that we should have an upper age limit of 60 years for heart valve surgery. Similarly, about 10 years ago we had an upper age limit of 65 years for coronary patients. However, we now know that patients of all ages, even those aged between 70 and 80, can have excellent results with coronary bypass surgery. This new treatment raises the question of age again. I think that one should not put too much emphasis on the chronological age of a patient but more on the biological age. We have seen many patients aged 70 or 75 with coronary artery disease who have not had an arteriosclerotic attack. We have also seen many patients with severe systemic arteriosclerosis who, in my opinion, are not suitable for coronary surgery or i.v. drug therapy in acute infarct. I think we should concentrate on the biological age of the patient.

HUGENHOLTZ:

I agree that the biological age is more important than the chronological age, but we know relatively little about this group at the moment.

VERSTRAETE:

According to your figures streptokinase treatment in Germany would cost about 300 DM and treatment with urokinase would cost approximately 1000 DM. This represents a 3.5 times increase in the bill for urokinase. It appears that urokinase is seldom used in Europe because of the cost, even though there are some benefits in using urokinase in terms of immunogenicity and some side effects are dispensed with. Are we making a drug that will not be used?

KLEIN:

Our department uses urokinase in about 20% of patients, and the remainder receive streptokinase. In general there are no definite criteria when deciding between the two drugs, except the possibility of side effects such as bleeding.

RUTSCH:

Dr. Klein, you indicated that the majority of patients with total occlusion of the coronary artery had complete infarction at 90 min after the onset of symptoms. Could you tell us the basis on which the data are derived?

KLEIN:

That was the Group A which showed no angiographically visible collaterals, but this does not mean that there was no collateral blood flow at all. If this is compared with scintigraphic studies and with the wedge pressure during PTCA, we can expect that half of the patients have at least some collateral blood flow which is not measurable by angiography. If there are really no collateral vessels and 20% of the patients do not dispose of any collateral blood flow at all, then we can make comparisons with animals that do not have collateral blood flow (i.e. rats and pigs). In pigs, for example, you can be certain that after 60 min of ischemia the infarct size cannot be reduced by reperfusion. Even after 45 min of ischemia you only can reduce infarct size within the septum, not in the free ventricular wall. It is already a transmural infarction after 45 min of ischemia. We should therefore separate patients on the basis of their collateral blood flow, because it has been clearly stated in hundreds of studies that collateral blood flow is the most important determinant of the speed at which ischemic myocytes die.

214

rt-PA – does this now mean thrombolysis for everyone?

R. J. Lennane

Boehringer Ingelheim Zentrale GmbH, Ingelheim (West Germany)

A somewhat clearer version of the title of this paper would be 'what is the final place of rt-PA likely to be in the overall therapeutic arsenal available to us for treating coronary artery disease?' (Please note that the term 'coronary artery disease' does not restrict itself to 'acute myocardial infarction').

Well, what do we know about rt-PA, what have we learned from this symposium, what can we take as established wisdom? I think it is fair to say that we all accept that it is an effective thrombolytic agent that opens coronary arteries. That seems

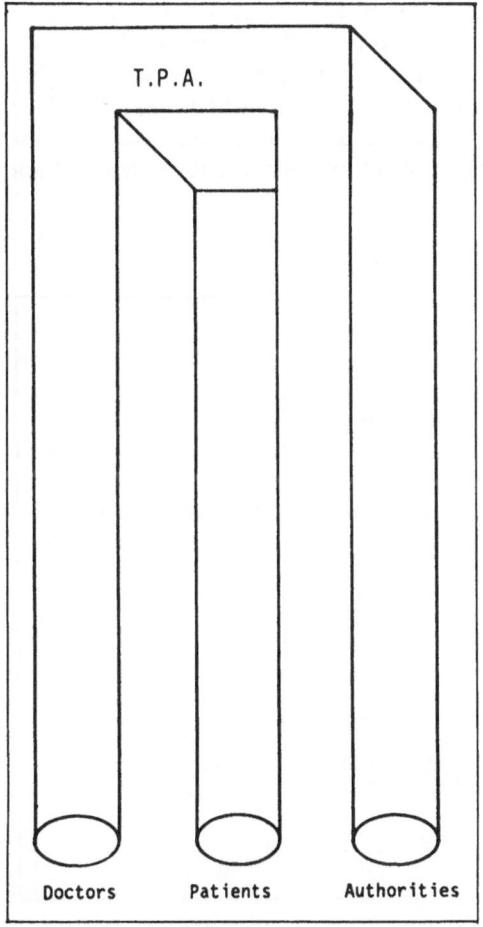

Fig. 1. A conceptual illustration of the difficulty in fulfilling all expectations

215

clear. And it also seems clear that this form of therapy is remarkably safe – it is really quite striking how few and how minor have been the side-effects in the studies reported so far.

The question arises, what more do we need to ask of it to really establish this therapy? What are our expectations? And when we discuss expectations we run up against the fact that expectations tend to differ according to who is doing the expecting.

Figure 1 illustrates in conceptual form the sort of thing that tends to happen: – however ideal your nice solid substance appears to be, it is still somehow not quite possible to satisfy everyone.

Notwithstanding these difficulties in getting things into perspective, what can we say about the place of rt-PA in cardiac therapy? Let us think about coronary artery disease for a moment in terms of a time spectrum as illustrated in Fig. 2. As can be seen from this fairly straightforward time-scale there are many points at which some kind of therapeutic intervention could be considered – in fact, given the current rate of progress in gene-technological research we might even be able to start one day at the very first point of all, and interfere with the genes. But as far as rt-PA is concerned we have concentrated until now on only one single point in the scale, namely the onset of an acute coronary thrombosis. I think that now we should let our thoughts run along the scale in both directions from this point, and consider what the place of rt-PA might be in unstable angina, for example, and in the prophylaxis of re-infarction in high-risk groups – questions for the future, of course, but concepts which might broaden our 'expectation horizons'.

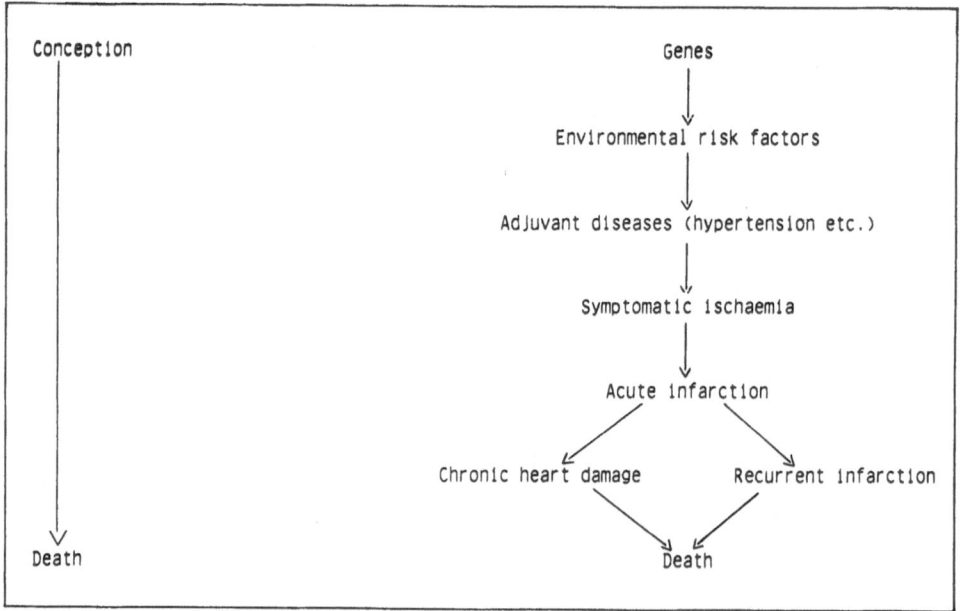

Fig. 2. Coronary artery disease viewed as a time continuum with multiple potential points of therapeutic attack

216

Now I would like to alter the emphasis and examine the place of rt-PA in the current gallery of thrombolytic agents available. (In other words I am retitling this paper: 'Thrombolysis – does this mean rt-PA for everyone?') We learn from the data presented at this Symposium that rt-PA is a more effective lytic agent than streptokinase, and it is remarkably safe. How far can we go in saying that rt-PA is *the* thrombolytic agent of choice available at the moment?

It is early days to be dogmatic about this, but certain points are worthy of attention.

1. Repeated dosing should be possible. Although not yet part of a routine clinical protocol the use of repeated doses of rt-PA is unlikely to be hazardous as careful searches for antibodies in the blood of patients receiving rt-PA have shown negligible antibody formation (unlike the difficulties encountered with streptokinase).

2. The ease of administration (simple i.v. infusion) and the lack of disturbance of systemic haematological parameters obviate the need for elaborate and expensive laboratory and angiography facilities.

3. Its safety and ease of administration suggest that it could be administered in the ambulance or even before the patient leaves his own home, with a consequent improvement in the critical interval between onset of symptoms and successful lysis.

I might also mention the recently published work of Sobel et al. (1) using intramuscular doses of rt-PA in rabbits: if this became feasible in patients it would of course revolutionize the ease of administration – but that is still only a gleam on the horizon.

Leaving these rather speculative areas, I will turn to practical matters, that is, regarding rt-PA from the point of view of its current availability and eventual cost.

To take availability first, I should start with the reminder that the very first use of rt-PA in a clinical trial in humans was only a very short time ago – in February 1984 to be precise! At that time there was only a very limited amount of rt-PA available. The method of manufacture, using techniques of recombinant biotechnology, was established in the laboratories of Genentech Inc., San Francisco, but at that time was capable of producing only relatively small amounts. It is true to say that in the first series of European trials we were living a hand-to-mouth existence, with small amounts of rt-PA being shipped across the Atlantic to us only just in time to keep the trials running. It was exciting, but somewhat insecure.

Happily, the situation is considerably changed. The manufacturing process for rt-PA has been scaled up, and the current availability is such that we have a much freer hand in designing a wide-ranging clinical trial programme. Nevertheless it is only fair to say that our prodigality in 1986 will still be limited to those investigators whose protocols, as judged by the Steering Committee of the European Study Group for Recombinant t-PA, really do make an important and substantial contribution to the overall development programme.

Now I come to the question of cost. There are two points to be made. Firstly, rt-PA is not and never will be cheap, for the very simple reason that making it is very difficult and complicated. For technical reasons it cannot be made in bacterial cell cultures. It can only be made in mammalian cell culture systems, which means that the conditions under which the cells grow, reproduce and are maintained and harvested require a very complicated, labour-intensive process, using expensive reagents, and so forth. So there is a basic manufacturing cost which is beyond our control at this time.

Secondly, if the question were asked 'what will be the cost of one rt-PA treatment for one patient' I would have to say that I do not know. No reliable estimate of the final price of rt-PA when it actually appears in the market-place can be given (although it will not be horrific). But even if it should cost an apparently high price (perhaps in comparison with streptokinase) its price should not be looked at in isolation, but one should consider the financial savings implicit in reduced morbidity, reduced need for elaborate investigational procedures, and reduced hospital stay; to name but a few related costs which it is only fair to take into account.

Finally, there is one matter which has not been mentioned at all, and I think it should be. When we have a difficult and complex project such as the development of rt-PA it is nice to have a patron saint. Of the possible candidates for the job of 'patron saint of thrombolysis', one front-runner stands out. I refer to St. Januarius, the Patron Saint of Naples. A small amount of his blood, preserved in a vial in Naples cathedral, miraculously liquefies twice a year. So if anyone knows all about thrombolysis it is St. Januarius, and I take the liberty of commending our project to his protection.

Reference

1. Sobel BE, Fields LE, Robison AK, Fox KAA, Sarnoff SJ (1985) Coronary thrombolysis with facilitated absorption of intramuscularly injected tissue-type plasminogen activator. Proc Natl Acad Sci USA 82:4258–4262

Author's address:
Dr. R. John Lennane
Boehringer Ingelheim Zentrale
Zentralabteilung
Medizinische Dienste
6507 Ingelheim am Rhein
West Germany

What should be the future strategy?

S. Effert and M. Verstraete

1. S. Effert

Department of Internal Medicine I, Klinikum der Rheinisch Westfälischen Technischen Hochschule, Aachen (West Germany)

According to Norbert Wiehner, the creator of cybernetics, intrapolation is from God, and extrapolation from the devil. The study of the future is a difficult science. The short term predictions are almost always wrong, and the long term predictions cannot be tested. But when I remain near the present repetitions are unavailable.

The thrombolytic agent of the 1990s will surely be an intravenous preparation with high clot selectivity, despite the fact that all of the presently available intravenous thrombolytic agents have a lower success rate than intracoronary streptokinase. The agent of choice is rt-PA at this time; clinical data concerning pro-urokinase and other agents will soon be available.

Future scientific activity must concentrate on three central problems:

1. The selection of appropriate patients

It is well known that the ischemic tolerance data from animal experiments cannot be directly applied to humans, for example because of the marked differences in collateral circulation. A definitive time interval for the individual patient, within which thrombolysis is still worthwhile, has not yet been determined.

Despite efforts to gain time, thrombolytic therapy should only be started when an exact diagnosis on the basis of acute electrocardiographic analysis has been made. Thrombolytic therapy should not be performed in the ambulance during transport to the clinic, nor by the physician. Its effect in unstable angina and evolving infarction have not yet been determined by a randomized study. Therefore, with suspected diagnosis of acute myocardial infarction, patients should be admitted to a hospital as soon as possible. At present, thrombolytic therapy does not appear to be of benefit in small re-infarctions in the same area.

The problem of indications in the case of inferior wall infarction arises from the fact that on the basis of the electrocardiographic results it is difficult to estimate the coronary anatomy and the size of the ischemic region.

2. When should coronary angiography be performed
if non-invasive tests indicate successful thrombolytic therapy?

Most patients have high grade residual stenosis after thrombolysis which presents a considerable danger of reocclusion. For this reason, angiography with the possibility of an early bypass or PTCA should be performed promptly after thrombolysis, to ensure that the early success is maintained in the future. These patients apparently have the best prognosis, although the costs are a problem. However, the data which have been available so far are derived from selected populations.

3. Continuation therapy following successful thrombolysis

This problem follows directly from problem number two. A randomized study to compare the effect of early bypass operation or PTCA versus thrombolysis on reocclusion, left ventricular function, and mortality, such as started for instance in Mainz and like the third European rt-PA study which will begin in January of 1986, has been lacking until now.

2. M. Verstraete

Center for Thrombosis and Vascular Research University of Leuven (Belgium)

It is acceptable to propose that almost all coronary heart disease is the consequence of coronary atherosclerosis and that thrombosis is a frequent endpoint resulting in occlusion of a coronary artery and the onset of an acute myocardial infarction.

A long-range view on the matter should therefore be: how can atherosclerosis at its very early stages in the first two decades of life be prevented; such a program should not be delayed until the disease continues to progress silently for decades until the clinical symptoms begin. Such a badly needed prevention requires the identification with non-invasive methods of youngsters at risk and the development of an effective prevention program of atherosclerosis in safe ways and compatible with an enjoyable life in the modern world. Progress has been made towards unraveling these first two questions but even if they were solved, many individuals at risk would not be identified in time or comply with restricting habits of eating and smoking, another life-style and possibly drug intake.

The second but less satisfactory level of protection is to aim at a delayed progression of already existing atherosclerosis, even at a stage that is not yet clinically apparent. Unfortunately the major risk factors of increasing age, male gender and poor family genetics are unmodifiable. It is therefore a sobering conclusion that only a limited number of risk factors can be modified, including elevated blood pressure, raised total serum cholesterol, smoking, glucose intolerance, physical inactivity, and obesity.

In a democratic society the best prevention program can be recommended by friendly persuasion – not imposed. Therefore, there always will be patients who develop extensive atherosclerotic lesions involving the heart, cerebral and peripheral arteries. Can we then obtain an anatomic regression of atherosclerotic plaques? There is limited evidence that atherosclerotic lesions can regress with treatment in a variety of experimental animal models of atherosclerosis. Over-extrapolation of animal data to the human condition is dangerous and direct evidence of regression of anatomic atherosclerosis in patients is scanty; moreover, the technique falls prey to confounding variables of fibrin deposition, dilatation, spasm, camera angles, etc.

What will then the future strategy be to treat patients with acute myocardial infarction, the ultimate event of coronary atherosclerosis in a patient who did have the chance not to die suddenly? In addition to offering immediate support to the pump function of the heart and preventing arrythmias with pharmacologic agents, the major urgent aim is to reduce the size of the initial infarct. Pharmacologic agents like beta-adrenergic blockers and nitrates may be useful and it is also a reasonable proposition that lysis of an occlusive coronary thrombus and early reperfusion of the infarct-related artery may shorten the twilight ischemic state of severely affected myocardial cells.

As the time-interval between onset of clinical symptoms of acute myocardial infarction and coronary reperfusion to be successful is very critical and short, the future of thrombolysis will be in applying simplified thrombolytic regimens. To this end, coronary catheterization with its delay, risk and cost should be circumvented in favour of systemic intravenous administration of the thrombolytic agent. This drug should rapidly dissolve the coronary thrombus and be fibrin-specific in order to avoid a generalized breakdown of the haemostatic system and inherent bleeding risk. Furthermore, the thrombolytic agent selected should be widely applicable and safe and should not require specific laboratory monitoring. In my opinion, tissue-type plasminogen activator and probably also single-chain urokinase-type plasminogen activator (scu-PA or pro-urokinase) provide a promising approach, either used alone or in combination, in view of their potentiating thrombolytic properties. Moreover, it would be most desirable to develop thrombolytic agents which can distinguish haemostatic fibrin and fibrin in a thrombus and whose long half-life allows bolus injection. Such agents should also be safe when given to a patient in whom the diagnosis of myocardial infarction was mistaken for an acute pancreatitis, ruptured abdominal aneurysm or perforated gastric ulcer.

Even the ideal thrombolytic agent will not modify atherosclerotic plaques and stenoses and will leave a recanalized coronary artery at risk of early or late rethrombosis. Thrombolysis can at best "buy time" for the patient so that early angioplasty or surgical revascularization can be peformed in a patient with a smaller infarct and result in longer lasting improvement of left ventricular function.

Thrombolytic treatment will not solve the problem of myocardial infarction which will probably remain a major scourge, but may considerably decrease its toll in terms of morbidity and mortality.

Author's address:
Prof. Dr. med. Sven Effert
Innere Medizin I
d. Med. Fakultät d. RWTH
Pauwelsstraße
D-5100 Aachen
West Germany

Author's address:
Prof. Dr. M. Verstraete
Katholieke Universiteit Leuven
Department of Medical Research
Herestraat 49
B-3000 Leuven
Belgium

A short overview summarizing two significant studies from the United States on rt-PA

R. v. Essen

The first prospective, randomized, placebo controlled trial of intravenous recombinant human tissue-type plasminogen activator (rt-PA) was published in 1984 (1). 45 patients (35 male, 10 female) with acute transmural myocardial and angiographically-confirmed complete coronary occlusion were prospectively randomized, two to one, in the treatment of acute coronary thrombosis with intravenous rt-PA or placebo. Interval from onset of pain to randomization was 284 ± 99 minutes (mean $\pm$ SD). Each of 5 additional, consecutive patients was treated with a high dose of rt-PA for two hours. 25 of 33 patients (75%) receiving 0.5 to 0.75 mg/kg body weight of rt-PA over 30 to 120 minutes had angiographically proven recanalization within 90 minutes of initation of therapy (Table 1). Only one of 14 patients given placebo had spontaneous recanalization within 45 min ($p < 0.001$). 13 placebo treated patients were changed over to intracoronary rt-PA treatment (0.375 mg/kg body weight). 9 (69%) exhibited subsequent recanalization within 45 minutes. The level of circulated fibrinogen decreased by only 8% of baseline value after treatment with rt-PA. None of the patients treated with rt-PA manifested a depletion in the fibrinogen level to below 100 mg/dl.

Clinical responses to infusion of rt-PA were generally favourable. Two of the 50 patients (4%) died with left ventricular failure (on the third and fifth post treatment days). One of these exhibited no recanalization. The other exhibited partial recanalization 15 minutes after onset of infusion, followed by reocclusion 30 minutes later.

No haemorrhagic complications requiring transfusion occurred within the first 24 hours after infusion of rt-PA. One patient had an episode of gross haematuria within hours of rt-PA treatment, and two had gingival bleeding during infusion.

This was the first study in which rt-PA was used in patients. Therefore it was, in part, a dosage-finding study. The results obtained indicated that intravenous infusion of 0.5 to 0.75 mg/kg body weight rt-PA, had a high thrombolytic activity and caused recanalization in ¾ of the patients without compromising haemostasis.

Table 1

No of Pat.	Dose (mg/kg)	Duration of infusion (min)	Recanalization	Partial recanalization	No recanalization
14	Placebo	30–45	1	1	12
	rt-PA				
3	0.25	30	1	2	1
3	0.50	30	1	–	2
15	0.50	60	11	–	4
15	0.75	120	13	–	2

Early reocclusion occurred in approximately 20% of successfully treated patients but only after discontinuation of the rt-PA infusion.

This first study with rt-PA in patients suggested that intravenous administration of this agent offers considerable promise for thrombolytic therapy in acute myocardial infarction.

The next trial was published in 1985 (2). It was the phase I study of the *thrombolysis in myocardial infarction trial* (TIMI). Phase I was designed "to assess the relative thrombolytic activity and side effects of intravenous rt-PA and intravenous streptokinase in patients with acute myocardial infarction and angiographic documentation of an infarct-related total occlusion of the coronary artery". All patients had a base line LV and coronary angiography with the infarct-related artery studied last after administration of intracoronary nitroglycerin (200 μg). Patients with a less than 50 per cent reduction in the diameter of the infarct-related artery were not given thrombolytic therapy. The primary focus of this study was the status of the infarct related vessel 90 minutes after the start of the infusion (either rt-PA or streptokinase). Each patient was randomly assigned to receive simultaneously either a one-hour infusion of 1.5 million units of streptokinase and a three-hour infusion of plasminogen activator placebo or a three-hour infusion of plasminogen activator 40 mg, 20 mg, 20 mg in the first, second and third hour) and a one-hour infusion of streptokinase placebo.

From August 20, 1984 to February 5, 1985, 316 patients were randomly assigned to rt-PA or streptokinase. Patients were excluded if more than 7 hours had elapsed since the onset of chest pain, if age was above 75 and if there were any contraindications against the application of streptokinase.

26 patients were not treated (8 had less than 50 per cent occlusion, 9 became unstable and the study of them was terminated, 9 had either technical difficulties or were outside study parameters). Of the 290 treated patients, 76 did not have total coronary occlusion before drug infusion. Thus, there were 214 patients who had a total occlusion (Grade 0, see Table 2 for gradings key) of the infarct-related artery at base line.

Table 2. Definitions of perfusion in the TIMI trial

Grade 0 (no perfusion): There is no antegrade flow beyond the point of occlusion.

Grade 1 (penetration without perfusion): The contrast material passes beyond the area of obstruction but "hangs up" and fails to opacify the entire coronary bed distal to the obstruction for the duration of the cineangiographic filming sequence.

Grade 2 (partial perfusion): The contrast material passes across the obstruction and opacifies the coronary bed distal to the obstruction. However, the rate of entry of contrast material into the vessel distal to the obstruction or its rate of clearance from the distal bed (or both) are perceptibly slower than its entry into or clearance from comparable areas not perfused by the previously occluded vessel – e. g., the opposite coronary artery or the coronary bed proximal to the obstruction.

Grade 3 (complete perfusion): Antegrade flow into the bed distal to the obstruction occurs as promptly as antegrade flow into the bed proximal to the obstruction, and clearance of contrast material from the involved bed is as rapid as clearance from an uninvolved bed in the same vessel or the opposite artery.

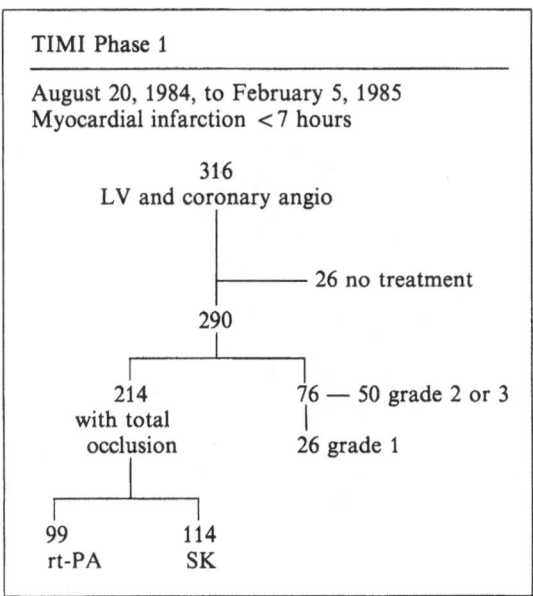

```
TIMI Phase 1

August 20, 1984, to February 5, 1985
Myocardial infarction < 7 hours

                    316
              LV and coronary angio

                    |_____ 26 no treatment
                    |
                   290
                    |
            _____|_____
           |                 |
          214               76 — 50 grade 2 or 3
       with total            |
        occlusion           26 grade 1
           |
      _____|_____
     |           |
     99         114
    rt-PA        SK
```

Fig. 1

99 were assigned to rt-PA and 115 to streptokinase. The mean time from the onset
of pain to the start of drug infusion was 287 minutes in the rt-PA group and 286 minutes in the streptokinase group (Fig. 1).

Of the patients with total occlusion, 59 (60 per cent) of those assigned to rt-PA had
90-minute reperfusion (Grade 2 or 3) as compared with 40 (35 per cent) of those assigned to streptokinase (P < 0.001) (Fig. 2).

If the 26 patients with grade 1 perfusion are added, there were 240 treated patients
– 118 given rt-PA and 122 given streptokinase. At 90 minutes, 78 patients given rt-
PA (66 per cent), and 44 given streptokinase (36 per cent) had recanalization
(P < 0.001) (Fig. 3). 19 of the treated patients died during hospitalization: 7 of 143
assigned to rt-PA and 112 of 147 assigned to streptokinase (5 versus 8 per cent).

There were no clear cut instances of fatal or central nervous system haemorrhages
in either group. Haematoma at the catheterization site was common, occurring in
43 per cent of the rt-PA group and in 47 per cent of the streptokinase group. Gastrointestinal bleedings were noted in 6 per cent and 10 per cent of the two groups,
respectively. Clinical reinfarction or extension, as assessed by recurrence of chest
pain and electrocardiographic and enzyme changes, occurred in 11 per cent in the
rt-PA group and 14 per cent in the streptokinase group (Table 3).

Although side effects were comparably high in both treatment groups and fibrinogen
levels, or levels of fibrinogen degradation products, were not reported, the authors
conclude that "an early recanalization rate of only about one third in patients with
total occlusion raises concern about whether treatment with an agent (streptokinase)
with substantial side effects is justified on a routine basis." They continue: "Although
the long term effects of rt-PA remain to be established, intravenous treatment with
this agent produced prompt recanalization in more than half the patients with

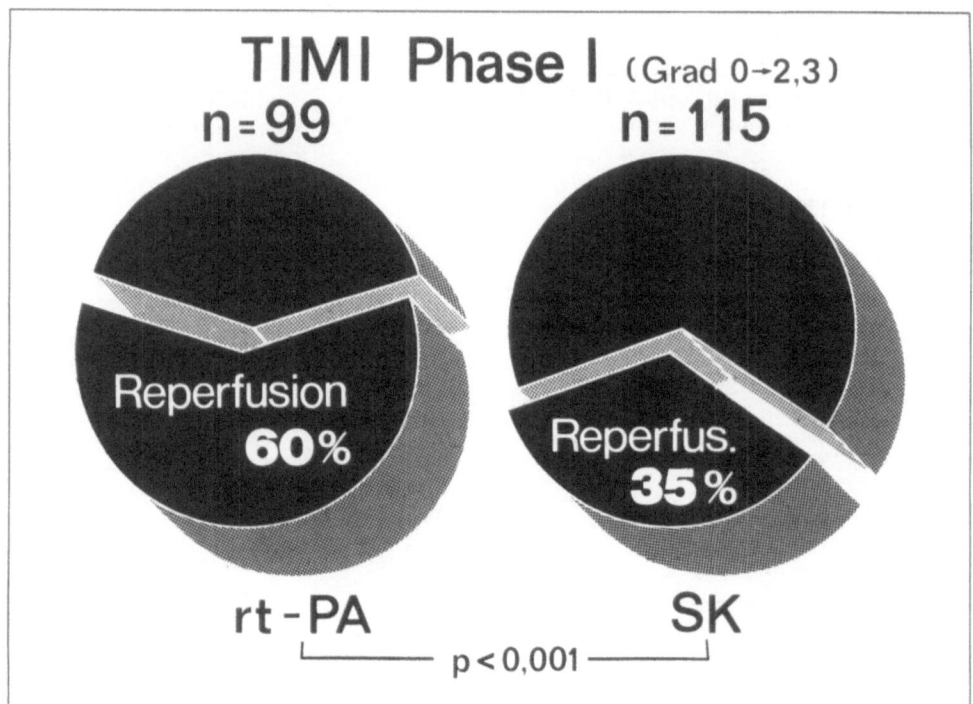

Fig. 2

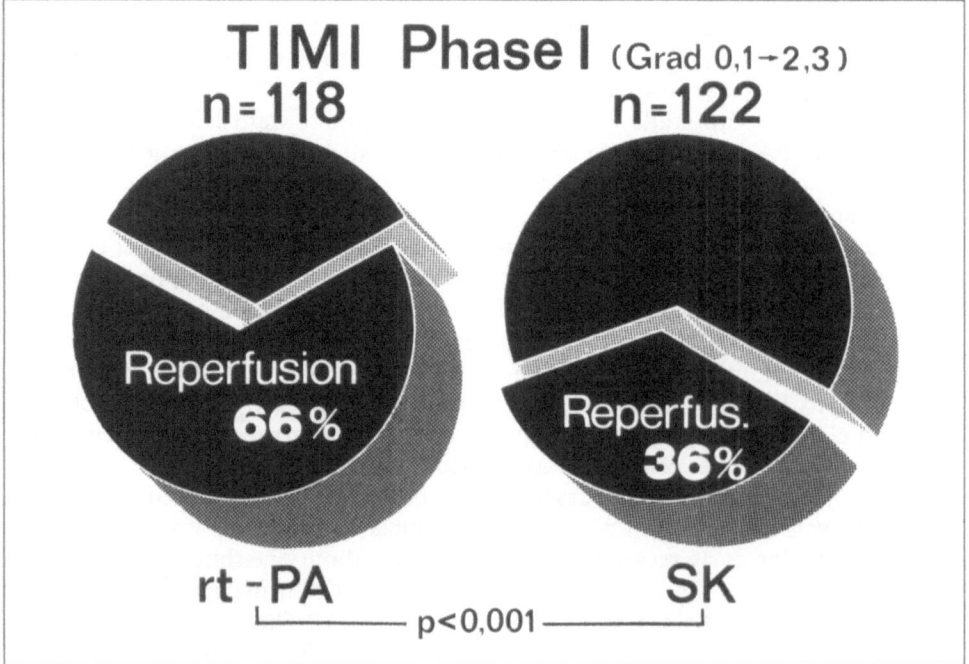

Fig. 3

Table 3

	TIMI-I	
	rt-PA group	SK-group
Hospital mortality	7/143 (5%)	12/147 (8%)
Extension of infarction or reinfarction	11%	14%
Haematoma at cath. site	43%	47%
Gastrointest. bleeding	6%	10%

total coronary occlusion; these results indicate that intravenous rt-PA does provide a change for favorably influencing the course in the majority of patients with acute myocardial infarction."

References

1. Collen D, Topol EJ, Tiefenbrunn AJ, Gold HK, Weisfeldt ML, Sobel BE, Leinbach RC, Brinker JA, Ludbrook PA, Yasudam I, Bulkley BH, Robison AK, Hutter AM, Bell WR, Spadaro Jr JJ, Khaw BA, Grossbard EB (1984) Coronary thrombolysis with recombinant human tissue-type plasminogen activator: a prospective, randomized, placebocontrolled trial. Circulation 70:1012–1017
2. TIMI-Study Group (1985) The thrombolysis in myocardial infarction (TIMI) trial. Phase 1 findings. New Engl J Med 312:932–936

Author's address:
Prof. Dr. R. v. Essen
Stiftsklinik Augustinum
Medizinische Klinik B
Wolkerweg 16
8000 München 70

CSI – A New Approach to Interventional Cardiology

Edited by W. MOHL, Vienna / D. FAXON, Boston /
E. WOLNER, Vienna

1986. 100 pages with numerous figures and tables.
Cloth DM 48,–; US $ 19.20
ISBN 3-7985-0694-9 (Steinkopff)
ISBN 0-387-91273-8 (Springer-Verlag New York)

Contents: Report of the international working group on coronary sinus interventions – The so-called "silent zone" of the coronary sinus – Inflow, outflow and pressures in the coronary circulation – Coronary sinus interventions: Clinical application – The promise and limitation of coronary venous retroperfusion: Lessons from the past and new directions – Synchronized coronary sinus retroperfusion current clinical perspective – PICSO status report 1985 – Retrograde cardioplegia: Myocardial protection via the coronary veins – 1986 – Technical aspects of coronary sinus interventions – Pros and cons-coronary sinus intervention vs. conventional therapy – CSI: Temporary support or long-term therapy.

CSI – A New Approach to Interventional Cardiology focuses on the clinical evaluation of systems such as synchronized retroperfusion (SRP), retroinfusion of pharmaceutical agents (RCSP) and pressure controlled intermittent coronary sinus occlusion (PICSO). This first volume of the series *Progress in Coronary Sinus Interventions,* with the latest contributions on the mechanisms, pathophysiology and anatomy of the coronary venous system, together with experimental results on coronary sinus intervention, thus provides the groundwork for further discussion, research and development in this field.

Distribution in US and Canada through Springer-Verlag, 175 Fifth Avenue, New York, NY 10010; for other countries through your bookseller or directly from Dr. Dietrich Steinkopff Verlag, P. O. Box 11 1008, 6100 Darmstadt/West Germany.

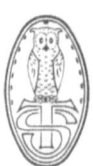 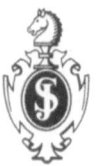

Steinkopff Verlag Darmstadt
Springer-Verlag New York

Controversies in Heart Valve Replacement

D. HORSTKOTTE, Düsseldorf · H. P. KRAYENBÜHL,
Zürich · F. LOOGEN, Düsseldorf (eds.)

1986. 360 pages. Cloth DM 120,–; US $ 45.00
ISBN 3-7985-0680-9 (Steinkopff)
ISBN 0-387-91269-X (Springer-Verlag New York)

Contents: Operative Treatment and Choice of Valve – Treatment after Heart Valve Surgery – Indication and Contraindication for Surgical Intervention – Operative Treatment and Choice of Valve – Diagnosis and Prognosis of Valvular Heart Disease – Indication and Contraindication for Surgical Intervention.

The implantation of prosthetic heart valves has a 25-year history. With this background experts in heart valve replacement gathered in Düsseldorf in May 1985 for an exchange of views, the results of which are presented in this volume. Opinions may be found on the diagnosis and prognosis of valvular lesions, indications and contraindications for surgical intervention, the choice of prosthesis, and operative and postoperative treatment.

This book is the first of its type to bring together all the essential problems of prosthesis heart valve replacement, which is still subject to controversy. The brief space of time between symposium and publication guarantees the topicality of this book.

Distribution in US and Canada through Springer-Verlag, 175 Fifth Avenue, New York, NY 10010; for other countries through your bookseller or directly from Dr. Dietrich Steinkopff Verlag, P. O. Box 11 1008, 6100 Darmstadt/West Germany.

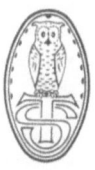 **Steinkopff Verlag Darmstadt**
Springer-Verlag New York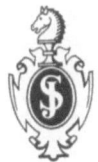